This warm-hearted, witty book dares you to cling to your neurotic symptoms, your depressions, your anxieties and your unhealthy relationships. From a wise counselor who has been helping people with problems for over twenty years, it is probably one of the most enlightening books you'll ever read and also one of the funniest!

Building on twists and paradoxes, Bill Little shows you how to *get rid of* problems by telling how to *produce* them. Sneak up on your troubles from behind and throw them all into hopeful perspective. Misery is an art—not just a state of mind. Learn it. Wallow in it. Use it.

Steer yourself toward an emotional precipice by snacking on Dynamite Sandwiches, playing Joan (or John) of Arc, being a Must-Win Loser. Live by the Pyrite (fool's gold) Rule. Or mess up your life with sundry colorful phobias, dependencies and addictions (including that classic problem-producer—alcoholism).

Looking for a mate? Reserve a place for yourself in a counselor's office by learning the fine points of poor mate selection. Enjoying a bed-of-roses marriage? Add some thorns by screwing up sex, thwarting communication, practicing creative jealousy. Still speaking to your offspring? Wall (don't bridge) the generation gap. Guarantee yourself a hostile household of mixed-up kids by screaming the impossible scream, expecting the moon and not being happy when you get it.

Healthy personhood can be just a book away; read *Self-Destruction Made Easy*—and drive yourself sane! Or give it as a present to any friend, acquaintance, relative or lover who could stand a little serenity or self-awareness, too. Satisfaction guaranteed—or double your problems back.

SELF-DESTRUCTION MADE EASY

BILL L. LITTLE
Foreword by Albert Ellis

PELICAN PUBLISHING COMPANY
Gretna 2006

To my family:
my wife, Gay, my daughters, Caron and Cheryl,
and my sons, Bill, Jr., and Russell

First published as *This Will Drive You Sane* by CompCare
   Publications, 1977
Published by arrangement with the author by
   Pelican Publishing Company, Inc., 2006

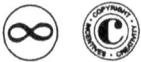

Printed in the United States of America

Published by Pelican Publishing Company, Inc.
1000 Burmaster Street, Gretna, Louisiana 70053

Contents

Acknowledgments

There are always many people who make possible the production of a book. I could never have had the time to put together even this brief work without the patience and acceptance of the people of Christ Memorial Baptist Church of St. Louis, where I have served as pastor since 1959. They are the kind of congregation that is conducive to health—theirs and mine. I hope their characteristically practical religion can be spread to many others.

Self-Destruction Made Easy is a result of a lot of ideas planted by various teachers and many friends. I owe particular thanks to my good friend Dr. Thomas W. Allen, professor in the Department of Counselor Education at Washington University.

I am grateful also to another good friend, my secretary, Sandra McWhorter, who has patiently typed and retyped the manuscript, as well as contributed helpful suggestions and personal encouragement.

I am indebted to Don Sparks, director of the Employee Assistance Program at McDonnell-Douglas Corporation, and to the people at the CareUnit at DePaul Community Health Center, Bridgeton, Missouri, for acquainting me with CompCare Publications. Diane DuCharme, CompCare's manager of publications, has been a teacher, co-worker and encourager extraordinaire.

I acknowledge all of the above and many of my counselees, students and members of a local CareUnit alumni group for their support and help.

It won't go without saying, so I'll say, "I thank God, who is the source of every good thing in my life."

Bill Little

Foreword

Bill Little's *Self-Destruction Made Easy* constitutes a rather rare work in the field of psychotherapy: one with a profound sense of humor, and one that employs jocularity to make many serious, sensible points. As he rightly notes, some well-known psychotherapists, such as Viktor Frankl, have espoused the use of humor in therapy and have demonstrated its good effects. Little might also have mentioned, in this respect, Frank Farrelly, whose technique of provocative therapy sometimes goes Frankl one better and takes clients' problems to hilarious extremes. Harold Greenwald, too, has espoused the use of jocosity and play in psychotherapy for a good many years and has given some fascinating talks and workshops on this subject.

I think I can, without any undue modesty, mention some of my own contributions in this respect. My first published book, *The Folklore of Sex,* partly consisted of a study of humor and sex, and also had its own highly jocular style—which, in those days of relative prudery, the prosexual critics heartily enjoyed and the antisexual ones hauled me over the coals for, seeing my witticisms as forced and inappropriate. I could say, of course, that the latter had no sense of humor! Anyway, nothing daunted, I continued to inject drollery into many of my other writings on sex and psychotherapy.

Even more than this, my therapeutic style, and that in which I conduct my public talks and professional workshops, has always overflowed with banter and jest—at least to my biased way of thinking; and not a few of my listeners, equally prejudiced no doubt, tend to agree with me. As for my regular group therapy sessions (which I still conduct on the scale of seven per week, since originating rational-emotive group therapy over twenty years ago), I would not exactly say that hilarity reigns supreme during these sessions, but it certainly tends to run a close second to the main theme of the groups: the teaching and experiencing of rational thinking.

Motivated by one of the basic tenets of RET (rational-emotive therapy), that of deliberate risk-taking in order to do one's own thing instead of remaining too beholden to the critical views of others, I finally made a uniquely humorous sally at one of the un-uniquely sober national conventions of the American Psychological Association in Washington, D.C. Before an unsuspecting audience of a thousand, I not only presented an enormously irreverent paper on "Fun as Psychotherapy," but I also illustrated my paper by singing, in my faded baritone, two of the humorous rational songs that I had recently composed.

Did all hell break loose as I belted out "Whine, whine, whine!" to the famous Yale Whiffenpoof Song and "Perfect rationality!" to the tune of Luigi Denze's "Finiculi, Finicula"? In spades! Deafening applause (for my erudition, of course); and during the rest of the convention, hundreds of souls, many of them among the horribly deprived who had not managed to get into the auditorium, kept greeting me in the hotel hallways and telling me what a great "talk" I had given. People who normally hated my guts and thought me a cold, overly rational fish, suddenly smiled on me benignly and told me how they now rated me as a great guy (and scholar). So humor really won that day—even among the sober psychologists. Sequel: the American Psychological Association received an unprecedented number of requests for copies of the tape recording of my presentation. Since no such recording existed, I had to make a special one later, as well as a cassette recording of several of my other rational humorous songs. (To get copies of either or both send seven and a half bucks to the Institute for Rational Living, 45 East 65th Street, New York, N.Y. 10021. Ask for my talk, "Fun as Psychotherapy," or my recording of "A Garland of Rational Songs.")

As my APA paper said, my own therapeutic brand of humor consists of practically every kind of drollery ever invented— such as taking things to extreme, reducing ideas to absurdity, paradoxical intentions, puns, witticisms, irony, whimsy, evocative language, slang, deliberate use of sprightly obscenity, and various other kinds of jocularity. Why do I emphasize humor so much in RET? Because we humans disturb ourselves emotionally largely by taking things too damned seriously—or by defensively going to the other asinine extreme and not taking them seriously enough. Instead of taking life with a bucketful of salt, and instead of mainly wanting, preferring, and desiring various things and relationships, we frequently demand or command that we get them. We insist that we absolutely *must* have them; and with this kind of *must*urbation, a form of behavior infinitely more pernicious than masturbation, we render ourselves disturbed and seriously defeat ourselves.

Humor can serve as an excellent antidote to our exaggerating the significance of things, taking ourselves and others too seriously, and perfectionistically demanding (and whining!) that we absolutely *need* what we *want*. And as I show in my APA presentation, rational-emotive therapists, including myself, frequently counterattack this demandingness in many witty and laughable ways. So does Bill Little in the present book. He shows how funny (or should I say tragicomic?) virtually all irrational, neurosis-creating ideas actually seem when looked at sensibly. He paradoxically overemphasizes negative thinking—so that readers can see for themselves how to do more positive kinds of thinking. He indicates the hidden gains people get from their nonsensical disturbances. He makes humorous mincemeat out of some of the grimmest symptoms of depression, anxiety, helplessness and self-loathing.

Actually, Reverend Little does a great job of making the reader think for himself or herself. For he so nicely presents the most dolorous sides of reality that he practically forces people to think of happier alternatives; and his entire book shows that humans have, if they only want to take it, an enormous amount of *choice* in their life circumstances—and even in the selection of their neurotic symptoms. Bill Little pointedly and wittily makes that choice crystal clear; so that virtually anyone who reads this book can appreciably widen his or her "free will" and intentionally *create* happiness and satisfaction instead of needless pain.

In my paper on "Fun as Psychotherapy," I listed ten major advantages of therapists using humor in their regular individual and group therapy sessions. As I read Bill Little's book, I see that, in its pages, as well as in the counseling sessions he cites in these pages, he has exemplified virtually all these advantages. For I find that: 1) His humor helps people laugh at themselves and thereby accept themselves with their vulnerabilities and their fallibilities; 2) It clarifies many of the client's or reader's self-defeating behaviors in a non-threatening, acceptable manner; 3) It provides new data and potentially better solutions, often in a dramatic, forceful way; 4) It relieves the monotony and overseriousness of many repetitive and didactic points which often seem essential to effective therapy; 5) It helps clients to develop a kind of objective distancing by participating in the therapist's (or author's) humorous distancing; 6) It dramatically and rudely interrupts some of the neurotic's old, dysfunctional patterns of thought and sets the stage for using new, more effective patterns of thinking, emoting and behaving; 7) It helps many people paradoxically think and act oppositely to their usual ways, thereby enabling them to do many things that they think themselves unable to do, such as behave unanxiously; 8) It serves as a distracting element that will at least temporarily interrupt self-downing and hostility-creating ideas that people use to upset themselves with; 9) It shows people the absurdity, realism, hilarity and enjoyability of life; 10) It effectively punctures human grandiosity—quite a disturbance in its own right!

I and several other psychologists who have investigated the function of humor in psychotherapy—and have ended up by enthusiastically endorsing it—have come up with these kinds of notable advantages of wit, drollery and paradoxical intention.

Bill Little, perhaps without making any serious study of humor in its own right, has beautifully applied these kinds of observations. With a rare wit of his own and the finest of therapeutic intentions, he has come up with a delightful book. I feel sure that it will prove very helpful to almost anyone afflicted with emotional problems.

Albert Ellis, Ph.D.

Institute for Advanced Study in Rational
   Psychotherapy and Institute for
   Rational Living
45 East 65th Street
New York, NY 10021

Introduction

Four things motivated me to write this book. First, during the past ten years while I have been doing therapy with people who have various emotional problems, I have occasionally observed a helpless group outside the therapeutic arena who seemed well-adjusted. Some of them were even happily married. Such people without problems know that they are out of vogue today. There are no television specials on how the well-adjusted person copes with life. The movies, television specials and feature articles are for people who are struggling with all kinds of problems. Problemless people cannot read with any real understanding the myriad articles on adjustment and mental health. They find themselves sitting quietly in corners when everyone else is talking about problems.

I am positive that inside they are a miserable multitude. If you are in this group, you do not belong. And everyone likes to belong.

There is hope for you! You, too, can have problems. Many of you have the innate ability and can learn quickly to develop problems serious enough for group therapy or even long-term individual psychotherapy. You neglected, problemless ones are my first reason for writing this book.

My second reason for writing this book is that I have observed how jealously people with problems guard their maladjustments. I have seen people use every imaginable technique, from denying and ignoring to open defiance, in order to hold on to their problems. It seems obvious that they would feel naked or at least foolish if they were living in the midst of all our solutions and were void of problems. Many of these poor souls just happened on to their difficulties and wouldn't know the first thing about PROBLEM-PRODUC-TION if they had to start from scratch.

It has been my conclusion that people hold on to their problems because they are comfortable with them. Many times they come to counselors to ask for help in living with their problems, not for help in getting rid of them. An alcoholic, for example, may have developed symptoms of depression, paranoia or something equally disabling. Such a person will ignore the fact that his or her symptoms are usually a result of the alcoholism. He/she just wants to be rid of the symptoms. In a situation like this, well-meaning, but naive, counselors will try to help the alcoholic by taking his or her basic problem away. Alcoholics who continue to drink do not want their problems taken away. They are comfortable with them.

It appears to me at times that homosexuals may experience similar problems to those of alcoholics. When they know they will be rejected by family and friends if they pursue their lifestyle, they suffer symptoms of depression and feel very misunderstood but still will not choose to opt for dealing with the cause. They are comfortable, and as long as they enjoy their misery enough to hang on to their problems, neither man nor God nor Sigmund Freud can take the problems away.

It seems apparent, therefore, that people want problems first because they like to belong and most of their friends have problems, second because they are more comfortable *with* their problems than they would be without them. People facing either of these two situations will be helped by this book.

There is a third very important reason for writing a book that will help people develop problems. Problems are most often useful to people. Emotional problems enable people to avoid hundreds of unpleasant tasks. People are helped to avoid facing the things they fear, and many people gain a lot of attention that would not otherwise be given to them. Therapists, seldom recognizing how useful emotional problems are to their owners, often accept the helpless concept preached by their clients. They rarely see how ingenuously people work at producing and protecting their useful problems.

The fourth reason for writing this book is a selfish one. I am astute enough to recognize that clergymen, counselors and psychotherapists need people with problems. Since I fall into the general category of those who need people who have problems, I feel threatened by people who have no problems. I'm much too far along in life to move into a new vocation so I want to help generate a market for my skills. It is sheer hell to have solutions and have no one to whom they may be marketed.

With such obvious needs on the part of patients and clients and with so many people depending on problems for their livelihood (thousands of us who, like vultures, traffic in the problems of others), why is there so little material available on how to develop problems? When so many people need problems, why so little work in this area? I have searched library card files, looked for cassettes, articles, anything! I have found precious little, if anything, that is really helpful. I hope now to contribute to the vast need for literature that will begin to fill a void in our present world. Of course, I suffer no delusions of grandeur at this point. I know that my work will be only a tiny seed. It will take at least a decade of research, isolating variables, accumulating indispensable statistics and perfecting techniques before real progress can be made. But where so much is needed, even a small start will be helpful.

In the interest of integrity, I should point out that at least two groups of people will not need the help that can be gained from reading this book: First, the therapists who engage in long-term therapy are usually well skilled in equipping people to hold on to their problems. A second group who will not need the help offered by this book will be the many clergymen who already are practiced at inducing guilt and generating problems for their parishioners.

In this book, I am offering you a selection of problems that should be adaptable to your unique situation. Of course, there is a remote possibility that just reading will not give you the problem-producing techniques you need. So, if you read this book and are still unable to develop even one problem of your own, go to a therapist who has no goals for you or who has a history of keeping patients for three to six years. And at the same time, it might also prove helpful to you to locate a church where the clergyman is known as one who is skilled in the art of guilt-inducement.

It seems clear to me that three groups of people can be helped by this book: 1) First, and perhaps most important, there are the lonely well-adjusted people who need help in developing at least enough problems so they feel that they belong. It is truly difficult for well-adjusted people to get that warm cuddly feeling of belonging in one of the most neurotic societies in the history of the world. 2) There are those people who already have problems and want techniques that will aid them in keeping their problems. Everyone seems to be helping the therapist. No one has come to the aid of the client who wants to develop skills for defeating the antagonistic therapist who is trying to take away his or her problems. 3) There are also the therapists who really want to understand their clients a little better. At the very least they may understand why their clients sometimes resist help so strenuously.

I started to write a book on solutions, but the market is already flooded with such material. When one cares as much about people as I do, he will find a need somewhere. I believe I have discovered that need. I offer this book first of all as a primary source of assistance to the heretofore well-adjusted, problem-free and all-too-often-silent minority.

Bill Little

Glossary of New Words and Phrases

Archeological Self-punishment—The practice of digging up past mistakes and/or bad experiences in order to make oneself feel miserable.

Basset Hound Syndrome, The—The habit or ability to take on the physical characteristics of sad-looking dogs in order to outwardly manifest inward sadness.

Bossophobia—The fear of bosses.

"But First" Syndrome, The—The practice of using the conjunction "but" in order to discount any positive feelings or experiences; e.g., "I'm kind to people, *but* they don't usually respond well to my kindness."

Circular Depression—Feelings of depression or sadness brought on by circular thinking. See "Circular Thinking."

Circular Thinking—Thinking that brings on circular depression. See "Circular Depression."

Double-bind Counterproduction—Combine any two or more of the four patterns of counterproductive thinking into a large economy-size dilemma.

Dynamite Sandwich—The explosive situation which ultimately results from packing negative feelings inside oneself.

Emotion in Motion—1. The ability to produce negative emotions while traveling, as in your car. 2. The ability to develop or sustain a feeling state while moving about, e.g., slouching and dragging your feet to sustain depression, as in applying the Basset Hound Syndrome.

Goal Ambiguity—The confused state of mental paralysis which results when one effectively blurs the focus in discussing problems.

Greener Grassing—The practice of thinking things are always better somewhere else or at some time other than the present.

I-told-me-so Syndrome—A pattern of thinking that produces your worst expectations, as in self-fulfilling prophecy.

John of Arc—A male Joan of Arc, i.e., a male martyr.

Mountain-building—The practice of stacking together many mole hills, or the ability to imagine mole hills as being larger than they really are.

Mulish—A Missouri word for extreme stubbornness.

Must-win Losers—People who, because they must always win, continuously focus on the next conflict or game, thus losing the pleasure of present achievements.

Negative Control—Producing problems to demonstrate the ability to solve them, e.g., deliberately crying to prove you can stop crying. The technique is an application of paradoxical intention whereby positive power is demonstrated by its opposite.

Negative Trinity—Fear, Guilt, and Rejection.

PAIN (*PA*radoxical *IN*tention)—The therapeutic practice of helping people to take control of their symptoms by directing them *toward* rather than away from their symptom; e.g., "You are feeling depressed? Go ahead and depress yourself."

Passive Communication—Talk with no action.

Phobiaphilia—The love of fear.

Postownaygut—An imaginative blend of Latin, Early American Pig Latin and German which means counterproductive thinking that says, "Wait for the good times that will come someday."

Postownaynichtgut—An imaginative blend of Latin, Early American Pig Latin and German which means counterproductive thinking that says, "The future isn't so hot."

Preownaygut—An imaginative blend of Latin, Early American Pig Latin and German which means counterproductive thinking that says, "The good old days were always better than now."

Preownaynichtgut—An imaginative blend of Latin, Early American Pig Latin and German which means counterproductive thinking that says, "The past was terrible and I won't forget it."

Principle of Perversity, The—Dr. Thomas W. Allen's way of describing basic human contrariness.

Pseudo-failures—People who deny their *success* and pretend or appear to have missed their goals when actually they have not. Such people are a genuine source of irritation to people who really fail.

Pseudopersecution—Self-inflicted persecution resulting from erroneous use of religious concepts. (Can be applied in non-religious people as well. In such cases the definition would be: Self-inflicted persecution resulting from erroneous use of *any* concepts.)

Pseudotrust—A phony state of confidence usually created in another person by lying to him/her. Frequently is started with the prevarication, "I want the truth."

Pyrite Rule, The—The fool's gold rule. "Don't care about others and they probably won't care about you."

Reverse Beasley Principle, The—The practice of taking on other people's problems as your own. (Internalizing; see page 3).

Screaming the Impossible Scream—A threat you have neither the means nor intention of carrying out; a form of Passive Communication, e.g., "If you don't sit down I'm going to cut your legs off!"

Sidetracking—The art of derailing discussion.

Snowballing—The practice of procrastinating when dealing with small problems until they grow into enormous problems.

Spouse Deafness—The ability to not hear your spouse, regardless of proximity of mouth to ear. Often results from passive communication.

Titanic Fear—The ability to believe that anything you fear must be worse than it appears to be. You only see the tip of the iceberg.

Trinity of Denial—A religious cop-out that leads to failure, hypocrisy and rejection.

Victim—One who not only *will* enthusiastically suffer for anything, any cause or no cause, but who *must* suffer for something and therefore is willing to suffer for nothing.

Volcano Effect—Emotional or physical explosions resulting from the excessive stuffing of a dynamite sandwich.

Volunteeritis—A form of avoiding relationships and responsibility manifested by donating service to less significant relationships and/or responsibility. A form of workaholism.

Want Power—A motivating drive usually mistaken for will power.

Water Route—The course of least resistance.

This Will Drive You Sane

Let's be honest. "Sane" does not mean "without problems." In fact, in our society it is insane to be without problems. It is abnormal and practically immoral to be able to say, "I don't have any problems." Even if it's true, you have to be insane to say it openly. Nobody likes a showoff, so if you have no problems, at least be quiet about it.

Most people have a few problems and can be helped to develop them more fully, while anyone can learn to have problems. This book can drive you sane, even if you are completely problem-free.

The good news is that problems seldom just happen. They are basically produced. With a little guidance, you *can* develop your own problem-riddled "sanity."

1

The Fundamentals of Problem-Production

Some people believe that problem-producing is more of an art than a science. This would mean that problem-generators are born, not made. I am sure, however, that any serious problem-seeker can produce the techniques that I am about to describe. If you really want to learn the art (or science) of PROBLEM-PRODUCTION, then read this chapter over and over until you have mastered the fundamentals.

Snowballing: A tremendously important technique which can change your entire life.

Many principles begin with myths, and the principle of snowballing is no exception. It seems that many years ago a wise man observed one he thought to be a fool. The foolish man was running down a snow-covered hill—with a small snowball rolling close behind him.

To the wise man it appeared obvious that the fool could stop, turn around, pick up the tiny snowball and throw it away. It was also obvious to the wise man that if the foolish man continued to run down the hill the snowball would grow and grow until it could literally mangle him. And that is exactly what happened.

Upon further reflection (wise men almost always reflect on things), he decided that the man may not have been a fool. Maybe he wanted to prove himself by overpowering a big snowball. Anyone could throw a small snowball away! Or maybe he was just bent on self-destruction and devised this magnificent, creative way to bow out.

The wise man never discovered the real reason but, being a real wise man, he shared the ideas with his kinsmen. Over the years they developed snowballing into a popular sport that has maintained its status to this very day. It is a sport not unlike the better-known game of risk called Russian Roulette.

The principle involved in snowballing is basic and essential to PROBLEM-PRODUCTION. If you stop and face problems when they are beginning, it is relatively easy to handle them. But for any person who really wants to develop problems, it is a mistake—a fatal mistake—to face problems early. Simply stated, the principle is: **"If you want to produce substantial problems in your life, you must avoid the temptation to solve them prematurely. In order to permit little problems to snow-ball, you must use every avoiding tactic known to mankind in order to permit your problems to get a firm foothold."**

One simple and very practical application of snowballing is practiced by many people prior to the income tax deadline in this country. They tell themselves to wait until a more convenient time before putting together the materials necessary for filling out the old familiar income tax forms. They avoid the temptation of putting records in convenient places, thus virtually assuring themselves of panic when income tax time comes closer and closer. What could have been a simple process, through record-keeping and filing, becomes utter chaos to the snowballer.

The concept of snowballing is mentioned early in this chapter because it is useful in the development of other techniques.

Snowballing is a sophisticated term for procrastination. It can apply to all areas of human life, including physical health, decision-making in business, religion, politics, home life, mental health, marriage and personal adjustment.

The best snowballers practice a simple rule: "When you think it is past time to do something about a problem—wait a little longer."

The Reverse Beasley Principle: The opposite of a problem-solving technique developed by a close friend of mine named Rod Beasley. I call his method "externalizing" or "the Beasley Principle."

Externalizing is the ability to permit other people to assume the responsibility for their own problems. As we shall see, problem-producers are frequently willing to assume the responsibility for anyone's problems. Beasley seldom, if ever, accepted the responsibility for another person's problems.

I was riding with Beasley one day when he stopped at a four-way stop sign. We had barely paused at the stop sign when a man in the car behind us began blowing his horn.

I said, "Beasley, that fellow is upset."

Beasley said, "Bill, that is his problem. My problem is to secure this intersection before proceeding." (He was an army man, and he always talked like that.)

As we moved slowly through the intersection, Beasley, looking both ways, was still talking, "... horn-honking doesn't bother me—I'm used to noise. In fact, that fellow can eat his steering wheel if he wants—it is not *my* problem."

Obviously, Beasley externalizes problems using this technique. We can reverse the principle and formulate one of the most clever of all PROBLEM-PRODUCTION techniques. It is sometimes called *internalizing*. **No matter what happens around you, no matter what goes wrong, develop the habit of blaming yourself for it.** If you work at it intensively, you will succeed in lowering your self-esteem to a problem level in less than a week.

Practical application is simple. Suppose someone doesn't like you. If you're a skilled problem-producer, your first thought will be, "There must be something wrong with me."

You can worry yourself sick just trying to figure out exactly what it is that is wrong with you.

People may ask you to do so many things you can't possibly get them all done. Instead of cutting back the number of activities and learning to say no, the effective problem-generators begin wondering what is wrong with them that they can't do everything they *should*.

Learn to say "That is my problem." Reverse the Beasley Principle. Internalize! Blame yourself!

Negative Focus: Or learning to look on the dark side.

It is impossible to overemphasize focus in PROBLEM-PRODUCTION. I have seen marriages thrown into gigantic pits of problems through the use of negative focus.

Don't let Norman Vincent Peale blind you with his positive principles. There is also power in negative thinking and negative focus.

An example will help to clarify the use of this technique. A few months back I was working with one couple very well-skilled in negative focus. Either husband or wife was able to pick up on the tiniest flaw in the other and twist it into a major criticism. They were so skilled at this process that I could never beat them at their game.

I suggested that they try to say one, just one, positive thing about one another. After a pretty good fight over who would go first she agreed to begin. It was beautiful! She pondered in silence for a full minute while he (and I) squirmed uncomfortably. Then, as if it was hard for her to speak, she said, "Well, he is a good provider, *but* he's a tightwad with all the rest of us." The *but* phrase was a gem, and it was uttered at a staccato pace.

For the moment he was wiped out. He was not, however, to be outdone. He was silent for a moment and triumphantly said, "Well, she is a clean housekeeper, *but* she bitches about every little thing left out of place." He flashed a quick winner's smile.

Like most good negative focusers, this couple goes through

4

a large portion of life "but first." This enables them to discount any positive quality they see in one another. Couples like this personify a quotable quote I attribute to myself: "Those who go through life 'but first' save face and lose all else."

What this couple did to each other, you can do to yourself. Find fault with everything you do. If you ever happen to notice something positive about yourself, quickly balance it by reminding yourself of a corresponding weakness. Focus on your weaknesses! Accentuate the negative. It works! You can generate anything from anxiety to depression through the use of proper negative focus.

Self-fulfilling Prophecy: This is certainly not a new concept, but it is so important in the creation and sustaining of problems that a few lines must be devoted to it. I sometimes call this the "I-told-me-so syndrome."

If you want to become a failure, predict failure. Say, "Oh, I can't do this" or "I know I'll never make it." If you expect bad things they are much more likely to occur. If you want anxiety you can have it. You don't even have to be a real failure. I have known some fantastic pseudo-failures who were as neurotic as real ones. The secret lies in what you keep on saying to yourself. "I am a failure" indicates failure whether it is true or not!

Some people say that you can make your dreams come true. Well, you can make your negative predictions come true also. Evidence of this fact can be found at any party. Just look for people who, having predicted they would not have a good time, are standing alone far away from the action. They will politely reject your invitations to join the group, then later bemoan the fact that "no one" would have anything to do with them.

There are myriad ways you can make creative use of self-fulfilling prophecy to produce problems. **You can be (or act like) a failure, suffer rejection, experience low self-esteem and even have accidents just by practicing negative expectation (not to be confused with unrealistic expectations).**

Unrealistic Expectations: Some of the most miserable people I know are those who have developed the knack for unrealistic expectations (this can be closely related or at least correlated with self-fulfilling prophecies concerning failure.) **If you want to be frustrated, then set your goals out of your reach.**

A counselee once told me that she was taking two college courses during her summer, learning to play the piano, caring for her three children alone (she is divorced) and looking after two sick relatives—all in addition to her regular work. To top it off she added, "And I won't be satisfied with anything less than 'A's' in my course work."

She is an expert. No amateur could devise such a schedule. I complimented her in a back-handed kind of way by confessing that I could add little to her goals. After a few minutes of silence (I use silence most often when I am stumped), I suggested that she might want to add more to her goals. For instance, developing the ability to leap a tall building in a single bound, outrun a speeding bullet or stop a locomotive with her bare hands. If she continues her present expertise at unreachable goal-setting she is assured of being a frustrated woman with low self-esteem. She will be a failure for years to come. At best, she will probably run into the side of a moderately tall building.

You need not limit unrealistic expectations to yourself. If you are married, you can produce some walloping problems by developing unrealistic expectations for your mate. For starters, expect your partner always to understand your moods and desires without your ever telling or revealing anything—always to like whatever and whomever you like—always to agree with you on every major issue—to give you undivided love, loyalty and attention and *never* to expect as much out of you as you expect from him or her. No one can possibly live up to all that. If you expect these things, you can confidently expect to be disappointed. You can also expect to totally exasperate even the most well-intentioned mate.

I visited a relative in the hospital recently. She was very upset because her husband had left her, alone and sick, while he went to the race track. Innocently I asked, "How did that happen?"

She said, "Well, he asked me if it would be all right, and I said yes."

"You mean you didn't tell him how you felt?"

"Of course not," she responded, "If he really loves me, I expect him to know how I feel." This is another clear illustration of unrealistic expectation.

The same basic principle can be applied to your relationship with your children. If you always set higher goals than they can reach, you can continuously widen the gap between you and them.

Apply this technique to any relationship. With a little effort you can become personally frustrated, a lousy mate, a poor parent and a friendless loner. As you can see, PROBLEM-PRODUCTION is not as difficult as many amateurs first suspect.

Goal Ambiguity: This principle can be stated as follows: **Commitment to a lot of things is less than commitment to one thing and thus will always leave you feeling uncertain about your accomplishments.**

Specificity is the hallmark of people who are solving their problems. Ambiguity is for the skilled problem-producer. It is not as difficult as it may first sound to you. Anyone who is sincere can blur his or her goals.

One effective way to blur goals is to set two mutually exclusive directions for yourself. If you are a housewife and you want to be *really* a devoted housewife, then add to *that* goal—the goal of developing a full-time career away from home, out of town if possible. You might even want to add school to your schedule, thus making it impossible for you to give all three goals top priority.

In addition to mutually exclusive goal setting you may practice the art of incompleting tasks. Never finish what you start. You may pursue a dozen goals without ever facing the danger of success and thus easily maintain the status of a

7

failure.* This is especially good for college students. Try this one on for starters: Begin in premedical school, but tell yourself it is too hard. Switch to law, then to psychology, to business, to education, to engineering. And if you run out of schools, start over. An efficient goal-blurring expert can remain in school for 10 to 15 years without graduating. Of course if you should be pushed into graduating, there is still graduate school. You can switch horses often enough to ride a herd and never get to the finish line.

Goal ambiguity also can be achieved through "greener grass" thinking. No matter what you are doing, tell yourself it would be better to do something else. No matter who you are married to, tell yourself that somewhere out there in the world is a more compatible mate. "Greener grassing" can keep you from achieving excellence in any job or can spoil any marriage.

Never clearly set a goal. If you blur your goals, you may reasonably assume that you will have more problems reaching those goals.

Phobiaphilia: In order to describe in technical terminology the tendency to take the coward's way out, I have simply combined the Greek words for brotherly love (philia) and fear (phobia). People who love fear as if it were a brother will always take the coward's way out. Those who have the most lingering problem-oriented lives seem to have an undying love for fear. They shy away from any decision-making that requires courage. Their guiding rule seems to be **"Never do anything that stimulates fear."** So, again learn from the experts!

To hang on to the problems you are generating by applying these basic principles you will need to develop a love for fear (phobiaphilia).

---

*Failure can be defined in any way that pleases you. One of the most convenient definitions for failure is "not reaching your goal." You can therefore set goals that cannot be reached and thus assure yourself of being a failure.

It is important to remember that when two courses of action present themselves to you, you must always take the course of *least resistance*. I have found that less resistance produces less fear.

Through my experiences in counseling, I have learned that key phrases help to solidify bad habits. Catchy nomenclature gives me a peg to hang my concepts on. I can say things like, "Take the water route." (Naturally, this is the course of least resistance or the coward's way out.)

I find that most of the time this course creates great problems for me in the future. It is easy, truly easy, to develop this habit. It enables one to avoid, temporarily, the responsibility for doing things that are difficult. A good slogan might be: "The easy I will do tomorrow; the difficult I will put off forever."

You may wonder how such an easy habit can help you develop problems. One illustration will help. A person in high school is often faced with a decision concerning whether to study or watch television. Most often the course of least resistance is watching television. Surely you can see how quickly this will produce serious problems for the student.

I suggest at this point that you take a break from reading and meditate on ways that you can apply this principle in your own life.

The Pyrite Rule:* Stated simply this rule says, **"Never give a damn about others and others will stop caring about you."** Reject others and they will reject you. This is an iron-clad rule in social relationships. It will surely bring about aloneness, which easily evolves into severe loneliness.

It seems to me that very few people understand the basic premise of the Golden Rule. The Golden Rule was given as a guide to social relationships. The basic principle is that we are to think of the good we would like to receive and then try to see that others receive that same good. What sounds selfish is

---

*Please note that pyrite is fool's gold. Literally, this is the fool's golden rule.

actually extremely unselfish, because the simple fact is that we can never love others until we learn to love ourselves.

In the interest of integrity I must tell you that I have never been able to totally apply the Pyrite Rule to myself. I have trouble believing that I will be rejected. I have the notion that I am liked. When I meet anyone who claims not to like me, I suspect that it is because that person doesn't really know me. The good news concerning this weakness of mine is that it enables me to care enough about other people to try to help them. I am now trying to help *you* by suggesting that you do as I say and not as I do.Try to dislike yourself enough to apply the Pyrite Rule.

If we disallow the positive rule (the golden one) as being selfish and also lower our self-esteem by saying to ourselves that we are no good and that we deserve nothing good, this lets us view others in the same lousy way. For once you lower your self-esteem, it follows that you will treat others as if they have no more value than you think you have—a sure technique to bring about your own rejection.

Say to yourself, "I'm no good. I have no value. I deserve nothing good." This will enable you to extend your negative thoughts to others. *They* are no good either, and their rejection of you proves it. Set it up. You will seldom fail to achieve the desired results. You can guarantee yourself rejection.

The Pyrite Rule works in PROBLEM-PRODUCTION because we get from others what we give to them. If you apply the Pyrite Rule, you can achieve a great deal of loneliness for yourself very quickly.

Once you have produced a good case of loneliness for yourself, you can begin to feel like all the other maladjusted people. You, too, can begin to seek help and become a genuine problem person.

Conclusion: Now that you have a basic overview of PROBLEM-PRODUCTION we can move into specific areas of practical application. The fact that you understand a basic principle doesn't necessarily mean that you can make the transition to the real world. I want to help you move these principles into practice so that you can choose to mess up specific areas of your life.

2

The Art of Misery

Depression is a state of unhappiness usually characterized by lethargy. We begin with depressions because they have so many practical applications. At its more extreme levels, depression can result in a total withdrawal from social contacts, including family and friends. Depression may become so severe that it will be characterized by thoughts of nothing less than a cloudy, beautiful sunset illuminating a crowd of weeping relatives who are sorry now. On the other hand, depression can be used to simply feel too low to go about your daily duties.

I hypothesize, with many others, that some of the basic causes for depression are feelings of unworthiness or worthlessness ("I'm no good to anybody and my life has no meaning"); feelings of guilt ("I am a terrible person, I don't deserve anything good"); most deadly of all, repressed or unexpressed anger or hostility. Note that in all these things it is possible for a person to, in Albert Ellis' words* "Say some-

---

*One of the books I most often recommend to people trying to get rid of problems is *A New Guide to Rational Living*, by Albert Ellis and Robert Harper. This book, along with Wayne Dyer's *Your Erroneous Zones*, will provide a good foundation for problem-solving.

thing to themselves about themselves."

It is my own personal belief that, even though a small percentage of the cases of depression around us are caused by circumstances and/or physical problems, most cases of depression are self-generated. Thus, like most other emotional problems, a depression is useful to its owner and is generated by him or her.

Now that you have an understanding of general principles, let us get down to the nuts and bolts of using depression in specific areas of your life.

The techniques being described here were not the theoretical musings of psychologists or psychiatrists or of other amateurs. They are the practical and proven methods of the experts. I have talked to my most depressed clients in order to discover their secrets. It is a slight oversimplification, but basically the psychological tool I used in gathering this information was the question, "How do you depress yourself?"

Heed this warning! I know these techniques do work, so unless you really want to become depressed, don't try them. If you already have a tendency to be depressed, you probably won't even need to read this section, but you can *read* it without *doing* it. I am sure most of you would like to try at least a little depression.

Some people are surprised by the "how do you do it?" question because they've always thought of depression as something that "just happens to them." When they feel depressed they have learned to say, "I am being depressed." They could more accurately say, "I am depressing myself." Surely there are circumstances that lead to depression, but it is rarely possible for the resulting bad feeling to get a real foothold unless we cooperate. The very least we can do is snowball and apply our phobiaphilia.

When people refuse to believe* that they actually do depress themselves, I ask them to just be absurd enough to pretend that they want to be depressed and think of ways that

---

*In some circles, refusal to believe the therapist is called "resistance."

they could do it. No one has failed to give me helpful suggestions in response to this imagined situation.

Think about it! Even as you are reading this paragraph, thousands of people are depressing themselves. They use an almost endless variety of techniques, only a few of which I am able to describe in this chapter. The fact that you actually have the power to depress yourself is important to those of you who want a good case of depression. PROBLEM-PRODUCTION works easily here. You don't have to sit around and wait for depression to happen to you. You can get out there and generate a good case of depression for yourself.

I have explained why I cannot take the credit for the insights disclosed in this section, but none of my clients wishes to receive credit for these insights either. Some of these clients are still actively generating and using their depression. If I reveal their identities, their depression would lose much of its usefulness. I couldn't conscientiously do that to people like one woman I know who is using her depression to get her husband's attention and to pressure him into doing the things she wants done. She says, for instance, "I just don't think I'll feel like getting out of bed this week if that family room isn't painted."

One of the men who shared some of these insights is using his depression to keep his wife from going on vacations without him. If she leaves (which he encourages her to do because he wants her to know how cooperative he is), he begins to feel so terrible that he just can't hide it when she calls home. She always has to come back home to him within two days after departure or arrange for him to meet her on the vacation trip. It is the only way to help him overcome his depression.

One young woman has for 20 years used depression as an excuse to stay at home with her parents and to avoid the responsibility of getting a job. How could anyone expect a depressed person to move out on her own and assume the responsibility for working?

Another person uses his depression for comfort and

responsibility. I will tell you his story later.

Depression is most useful for avoiding responsible action. Who can expect depressed people to make decisions or face issues? Decisions will only make them more depressed.

Another of my authorities decided to give up her depression and go in for something less drastic. She has developed a nasty temper to help control the people in her life. She finds that it works just about as well as depression and doesn't leave her feeling so bad.

In order to enable my expert producers of depression to maintain their anonymity, I have combined their suggestions into the following useful techniques for developing depression.

1. Play sad music softly. There are exceptions to this (I know of at least one young woman who found hard rock music most helpful in depressing her), but most of my clients say that something soft and sentimental is best. Music also can be a good background for any of the other techniques listed in this chapter and can be used in connection with most of them.

In our section of the country (St. Louis, Missouri) many people use country and western music to help them develop depression. When they have too little time to watch soap operas, they have discovered that the same mood can be generated by listening carefully to the words of a good tear-jerking country and western song. People in a hurry, who just have to get someplace, may listen to these songs in their own cars. I call this depression-on-the-go or *emotion in motion*.

2. Turn the lights down low. Some people turn them off completely; others just dim them. On bright days, close the drapes or pull the shades. Dimly lit or dark rooms are much more conducive to depression than bright rooms. Obviously night time is best for producing depression. Your neighborhood bar can usually provide you with both the preceding conditions, plus serving you liquid depressants. The bar atmosphere is especially effective if you come in and leave alone. Remember this suggestion when you read technique number four in this chapter.

I strongly recommend that you take advantage of natural conditions. If it is a rainy, nasty, gray, cloudy day there is a natural darkness. The beauty of using weather conditions to aid in the production of depression is that on the deepest level of thought you can assume that even God is against you. Now that *is* depressing!

3. Focus on the negative. Think of all the bad things you can remember. If you can't remember any bad things, read a newspaper. You can always find something bad in the paper. In PROBLEM-PRODUCTION, focus is one of the most important of all tools. Learning proper focus puts you far ahead of the crowd. It might prove helpful for you to review the general technique of negative focus.

Remember the times you were treated unfairly or the times someone spoke unkindly to you. It will help you to write down your rotten experiences in detail. You can easily generalize from just a few specific cases. You can say to yourself "That's the way the whole world is. I am always misunderstood and mistreated by everyone."

Note the use of sweeping universalities such as, "always," "everyone," and "the whole world." Big things enable you to forget little specifics. It is much heavier to carry the whole world and everyone on your shoulders than just the one or two people actually involved. Repeat these generalizations over and over as you sit in a dimly lit room listening to sad music.

4. Be alone as much as possible. You will be able to give more complete attention to your negative thoughts if you are alone. Being alone sometimes helps one to verify any negative suspicions. "Nobody really cares about me, I'm here in the dark all alone." See how it works?

5. Remember all the bad things you have done. Surely most of us can remember at least one bad or naughty thing we've done. Perhaps we can even remember some downright evil, depraved act. For instance, I remember slightly exaggerating a dream I had when I was seven years old, I was a liar. I can accomplish this kind of *archeological self-punishment** without much effort at all, and I don't even claim to be an expert at depressing myself.

I also know that most people can dredge up a flaw or two, because I have never met a really perfect person. If you have trouble remembering your bad behavior, make up something. It will work just as well. Once you can zero in on something bad you've done, been or could have done or been, you can begin to generate guilt and thus depression.

Say aloud or think to yourself, "I am a terrible person. I shouldn't have done this or that terrible thing in my life."

Whatever you do, do not rationalize your bad deeds and *never* try to make restitution for any of them. Don't allow anyone to forgive you—for that would destroy the affective power of your deeds. This technique is so powerful that even a beginner can use it to produce guilt feelings and thus start moving rapidly toward real depression.

6. Remember all the good things you could have done. This technique focuses on sins of omission (sins from which you receive no pleasure at all). It is easy to make an endless list of all the potential good you have missed. Think of the books you could have written, the jobs you could have had, the opportunities you passed up, the people you could have helped, the souls you could have saved, even the fights you could have stopped. If you make a long enough list, you can begin to feel guilty and once again start moving toward the depression you are trying to produce.

7. Try the impossible. Set out to achieve a goal that is beyond human capability. You are a cinch to fail. Pause for a moment and ponder unrealistic expectations as described in the preceding chapter.

---

*This is the knack for being able to dig up bad relics from the past.

Failure, even to accomplish the impossible, can bring on intense feelings of worthlessness and, hence, depression. If you want to do well at PROBLEM-PRODUCTION, you *never* accept an approximation of your goal. "All or nothing" is the motto for the expert at depression. "I *never* do *anything* right. I'll *never* make it. I am a *total* failure." Again, note the use of universal words.

8. Refuse to admit feelings of hostility or anger. Certainly avoid expressing them! It is easy to repress hostility. You only need to say to yourself that you have no right to feel angry. There must be something wrong with you if you feel hostile. Refuse to admit or express such feelings.

Repression of hostility is the *most powerful* of all techniques for becoming depressed. Think to yourself, "I have no right to feel this way. I should not feel angry, but I do."

Refuse to express your feelings. Press them down. Hold them in. You will produce what I call the *volcano effect** and erupt into a fit of rage over some insignificant "straw." You will then feel guilty because of your incongruent overreaction or you will internalize your anger and feel miserable. Do not despair even if you happen to slip and express a negative feeling. You can easily develop guilt over your honest expression and quickly retreat to repressing your feelings once more. You cannot lose!

9. Associate with depressed people. Seek out as many depressed friends as you can find. It is usually easy to find depressed people, just check out any dark places!

In the unlikely event that you do not find a depressed person, you can get almost the same effect from the opposite extreme. Find someone who is unrealistically happy, a real Pollyanna. Such a person can make you sick in a hurry. I still think it is better to reinforce your depression and low self-concept by associating with fellow self-depressers. Then you can use old sayings to reinforce your condition. "Birds of a

---

*Pack enough unexpressed feelings together and you will blow up.

feather flock together." "Misery loves company." "It takes one to know one." (Just *saying* these old sayings can be depressing.) You are now on your way to genuine depression!

Here is a clinical example of these techniques as practiced by one of my depressed experts.

I recently talked to this man, who had twice made rather colorless attempts at suicide. He was terribly depressed, obviously an expert. I asked him how he depressed himself.

He said, "I don't know. Something just clicks, and then I'm depressed."

Not to be denied, I went on, "Well, if you wanted to be depressed what could you do?"

"Oh," he replied with sudden insight, "I could have an argument with my wife and yell at her a lot. That makes me feel pretty bad." (A cooperative mate can many times help us develop depression.)

"What else?" I asked.

He smiled, hesitated, then said, "I could miss work and cut class."

"Then what would you say to yourself about that?"

"Oh, I guess I'd say, 'I shouldn't have done that, I probably missed something really important.' Then I feel very bad." Again, he paused, glanced sideways at me, and went on. "I've always thought it was the other way around. I thought I got depressed, then missed work and class. Are you telling me it is not that way?"

I would not fall for it. "No, I'm not telling you anything, just asking." The look on his face revealed that he had been discovered. I really felt a lot of sympathy for him. What had I done? I had revealed his technique to him and thus made it less useful. I really doubt that these two techniques will work as well for him in the future, but I figure that anyone with his ingenuity will devise new techniques. He was so insightful that I suspected he might know even more. Few people are aware of the value they receive from their problems, but I thought he might be, so I asked, "What do you accomplish by being depressed? Do you think you get anything out of it?"

It was as if the answer was on the tip of his tongue. "I don't have to reach my goals in life if I am depressed. That's on the negative side. On the positive side, I feel like I'm in a comfortable corner—very secure ..." He looked at me after pausing and said, "Hey, are you saying I use my depression for this?"

"I'm not saying anything, just asking." Obviously I was beginning to feel bad by this time. I had inadvertantly assumed that he wanted to stop being depressed. I had come dangerously close to taking his techniques away from him. Thank God, the session was nearly over.

I have two reasons for sharing this clinical example with you: 1) This client generated his own depression. You can generate your depression too. 2) He used his problem. You, too, can use your problems.

3

Depression: Let It Show

No doubt some readers will not be satisfied with general principles that produce feelings of depression. Some of you are such perfectionists that you will not be satisfied to simply *feel* depressed. You will want to develop this science or art of depression so fully that not only will *you* know that you are depressed, but *anyone* who sees you will know it.

You are among the faster learners in PROBLEM-PRODUC-TION because you are highly motivated. You will not be satisfied until you are depressed inside and out. You are not only among the most likely long-term depressees—you may well become a depressor. You are a potential carrier of depression. Only perfectionists can reach this ultimate state and become carriers. Depression can be contagious.

The suggestions that follow are not simply hypotheses. Like the previous suggestions, these are techniques tried and proven by experts. I will begin with general external appearances and move inside from there.

1. Getting Into the Basset Hound Syndrome:* I recommend

---

*Special note to dog-lovers: Basset hounds are cute dogs, but they were not designed to be people. Of course, if you want to be upset by what is not meant as criticism of dogs, go ahead. But please refer to my chapter on negative focus for guidance.

that once you have started your trip toward depression, you allow yourself to really get into that depression physically. Let your outward appearance transparently reveal your inner gloom.

Imagine that you are a humanized basset hound. Visualize yourself as a poor whipped basset puppy. If you can put a picture of the sad-eyed little fellow on your desk, mirror or refrigerator door, it might help.

Let your body get into the mood. Stoop, droop, slump, slouch and sag wherever your muscle control will permit. Feel your eyes droop. If you really get into this with your total being, you may even feel your ear lobes sagging.

Advertising helps so let your depression show through your sloppy appearance. Some people are able to allow personal hygiene to slide, too. You can try it. Simply stop washing your hair and brushing your teeth and start to wear wrinkled old clothes. When you feel lousy inside, let the whole world know.

It will help if you walk slowly. You should even drag your feet when possible. Remember that snappy walking or good posture fights against depression. I put it in these easy-to-remember words: Poor posture poops you out. (This is an alternate form of emotion in motion.)

2. Wear a frown: Frown and frequently the world will snarl at you. *Never Smile!* It is hard to convince those around you that you are depressed if you permit yourself to smile.

If some insensitive person says something hilariously funny and you inadvertantly smile, quickly squelch it. Remember that basset hounds seldom appear to be smiling. If you are going to be depressed, look depressed.

3. Sound depressed: Talk in a low monotone or a basic whine. (Whining is more effective if you can get into a nasal tone or twang.) When you remove the inflections from your voice, you automatically begin to feel worse. Even if you are not genuinely depressed, this technique will make you sound depressed. In addition to sounding depressed, you will become irritating to the people who listen to you talk. With any luck at all, you'll soon have most people doing their best to get away from you. This will give you a sense of real rejection, which can lead to real feelings of depression.

So do not yield to the temptation to change the pitch or add color to your voice, lest you spoil the whole effect for yourself and for others. Do not take this lightly. It is no easy task.

Many occasions can cause you to slip and forget yourself. You may see something exciting—say, an accident on the highway. You may be tempted to raise your voice and exclaim something like, "Oh, my lord, look at that, twelve cars and a..." Don't do it. Control yourself with a low grunt or a whining statement such as, "That's the way this stupid world is."

Monotones or whining and bland facial expressions fit together hand in glove and certainly aid in the achievement of depression.

4. Avoid eye contact: Look at the floor or stare aimlessly into the distance. People will suspect you of being reasonably well adjusted if you maintain a fair amount of eye contact with them.

Keep looking down whenever possible. Not only will you be sure to see a lot of dirt, but your concentration will never be broken by the intrusion of faces and things.

I have learned from depressed clients, who testify that depression is aided by avoiding eye contact. One young girl refused to look at me. It was as if her gaze was glued to the floor. I finally broke into her line of vision by lying on the floor and looking up into her eyes.

At first she resisted by moving her stare slightly away from me to other spots on the floor. I would not capitulate. I moved to the new spots. She smiled a meek, loser's smile and said, "All right, if you're going to do that, get in your chair. I'll look at you." Contact was established. What is the moral of this story? If you want to hold on to depression, never allow the contact to be established.

5. Try circular thinking: You can look depressed, sound depressed and think depressed. Circular thinking is closed thinking. It can be achieved by almost anyone. I'm sure you can do it. All you have to do is figure out two or more ideas that lead to each other.

One of my clients devised this magnificent circle: She is unmarried and tells herself that there is little hope that she will ever find anyone to marry (one of the few turns of fate that she feels would bring her happiness). She also has what she calls high moral standards, so having sex generates deep feelings of guilt. In a moment of weakness, she yielded to her natural inclinations to have sexual relations and discovered that she temporarily felt better. That is, until the guilt moved in. Now she is trapped in a vicious circle. She decides to have sex. Then, because, as I told you, she is highly moralistic, she feels guilty about sex without marriage. Her guilt makes her feel depressed, and in order to get over her depression, she has sex. Sex makes her feel guilty, so she becomes depressed and on and on or round and round she goes. Depressing, isn't it?

You can imprison yourself inside your own neat circles by adding to your existing feelings of depression anything that makes you feel guilty. Tell yourself that it is essential for you to do the guilt-inducing thing—whatever it is—in order to feel better. You are on your way.

Use any appropriate action to complete the circle—eating (if you are a dieter), drinking booze (if you are a problem drinker or an alcoholic), spending money, working compulsively, gambling, etc. There is always something you can indulge in to make yourself feel guilty. Having done this, you have locked yourself into the golden circle of depressive thinking.

6. Don't be afraid to use other people. Choose your friends carefully. If you find someone, anyone, who will laugh at you when you feel bad or call attention to how terrible you look, cherish that person. Spend as much of your social* time with that deprecating person as possible.

In the absence of an insensitive friend, a spouse or other family member can help. Listen for their most insensitive statements, and never forget those words.

Hear now the temporary conclusion to the whole matter concerning depression. First, use general techniques to produce depressed feelings, then look depressed, sound depressed, think in depressive circles. Spend time with people who reinforce the whole process. Application of this approach is a sure sign that you have become an expert at depressing yourself as well as a highly contagious carrier of depression.

---

*Spend your social time wisely. It is best not to spend much of your time socially anyway, because that is self-defeating to people who want to be depressed. Keep your social contacts to a minimum.

4

Problem Development:
Guaranteed Methods

Dynamite Sandwiches

It is helpful to be able to conceptualize clearly the principles we use. A visualization is worth 872 words. One of the basic principles in developing problems is what I call the volcanic effect, or the Dynamite Sandwich. Now this is a principle that you can *see!* Let me explain.

This visual and effective way to generate problems for yourself involves repressing your feelings. Little feelings that have a very small, if any, noticeable effect on you or the people around you can be packed together until they become explosive.

Well-adjusted people, perhaps like you were before you began studying this book, learn to express feelings effectively. They express themselves at what some assertiveness trainers call the minimum level of effective communication. What this means is whenever they begin to feel irritated, they simply tell the person or persons with whom they are becoming irritated that they are feeling irritation at whatever is happening or being said. When there is a major problem they react at an appropriately higher level. This means that their reactions match their feelings in scale.

If you adopt that behavior, your chances for producing problems are greatly reduced. To become effective at problem-producing, you must learn to repress feelings until you can no longer possibly conceal them. In other words, you learn to explode. The technique is tried, proven, and guaranteed to bring immediate results! It is impossible to predict beforehand whether your blow-up will be outward or inward. It really doesn't matter—the important thing is that there will be an explosion.

Repressed or unexpressed feelings can explode inward and generate depression, indigestion, headaches, ulcers or even heart trouble. Or—they can explode outward and generate violently hostile reactions from your wife, husband, son, daughter, other family members, any close associate or some equally innocent bystander.

Think of it this way. Imagine two slices of bread lodged inside you. One is wedged at the top of your chest near the base of your throat, and the other sits an inch or two lower down. The distance between them varies depending on your tolerance level. Each time you discover a feeling and refuse to express it, you pack a little piece of filling between the two pieces of bread. Like anything else, your dynamite sandwich will soon be stuffed to capacity. The next repressed feeling will cause one slice of bread to explode.

If the explosion goes up and out, you may have a temper tantrum, wildly scream or tear through a room breaking things. If the explosion shatters the lower slice, you will have internal reactions like stomach problems, migraine headaches or perhaps even a good case of depression.

Remember the chapter on "The Art of Misery" where you learned (if you didn't already know it) that the cause of depression is unexpressed hostility or unexpressed negative feelings, such as anger? If you have been skilled enough to begin generating depression, apply all the other principles from "The Art of Misery" for a genuinely deep depression.

My other name for the Dynamite Sandwich is the *volcanic effect* because the boiling feelings you store up are bound to erupt eventually through the surface. This is a fool-proof technique, and anyone can master it.

You can make any kind of sandwich that suits your taste. You can fill it with unexpressed feelings about sex and have a sexual sandwich, a sexual explosion. You can stuff the bread with feelings about in-laws, children, employees, teachers, students, politics or cars or any one of hundreds of things.

An ingenious variation is the smorgasboard sandwich. Pile in feelings from any number of situations indiscriminately. This variation can be used to baffle a psychotherapist for weeks.

Couples produce the Dynamite Sandwich effect by refusing to deal with problems. It is similar to snowballing. I know of couples who have saved up or repressed their feelings long enough for complete break-ups. If you refuse to express feelings or deal with problems for a period of months or even years, you will literally build up enough pressure to blow your relationship apart.

One woman, whose husband came to me for help had "suffered in silence" for seventeen years. She crammed the sandwich full, then she packed her clothes and left. He didn't even know the bread was loaded until the explosion occurred. They decided against divorce, so she had to stop suffering in silence. When she wants to develop another problem, all she has to do is start packing her feelings away again. It will not take seventeen years next time!

Anyone can be a sandwich chef. Just stop expressing your feelings, or never start expressing them. You'll have at least a small pop within a few days, and, with a little effort, you'll soon be the parent of a mighty boom.

Becoming "Must Win Losers"

Well-functioning people are not threatened a great deal by losing a game or even an argument. They either chalk it up to experience or just ignore the defeats and move confidently onward.

Weak and insecure people must win—or so they tell themselves. It doesn't matter whether they are arguing about politics, religion or playing a game of checkers. They become overwhelmed at the hint of defeat, and at the same time they are never secure with their victories because there is always another challenger ahead. After all, everyone guns for the fast gunner.

They are masters at "self-talk" (lay people frequently call this "talking to yourself"). They say to themselves, "I must win or I'll become a laughingstock. People will think I am a pushover. They'll see how weak and inept I am." People who talk to themselves like this always have to be winners, and, since that is impossible, they live in constant fear and always carry instant anxiety on their overloaded shoulders. They are consistent losers—even when they win—thus they are "Must Win Losers."

This problem willingly lends itself to marriage relationships and to parent-child relations. It is used in employee and employer relationships, teacher-student relationships and in any situation involving people. Anytime two people are involved in interpersonal relationships, insistence by either one that he or she must win will assure both of them of losing. That is a problem produced by "Must Win Losers."

You can become a "Must Win Loser" by repeating to yourself the inner dialogue stated above. It may take two or three hours, but practice can make you imperfect when you genuinely put yourself into it. Self-discipline is essential to good PROBLEM-PRODUCTION.

Burn Yourself at the Stake

You can become a Joan of Arc or a John of Arc, if you are willing to spend a little extra time talking to yourself. Martyrs are some of the most skilled self-talkers in the world. All you need is opportunity, and in this case it is clearly true that those who seek shall find.

Mothers can overburden themselves with everyday household chores. Say to yourself, "No one really cares about me. All they want is what I can do for them. As far as my children are concerned, I am just a slave."

Fathers can use the same approach. It is easily adapted by either spouse. "I work my fingers to the bone, and no one really cares. Everyone uses me and that's awful. I am never appreciated."

As in all areas of self-talk, truth is irrelevant. We make our own "truth" by what we do and what we say to ourselves about what we do. This process can be applied socially, in PTA, in church, at work, at home, at school, and even in the bathroom. You can easily set yourself up to be overburdened. Begin immediately to tell yourself "how awful life is."

Burning yourself at the stake is not only helpful in generating bad feelings in yourself. It quickly disgusts the people around you and produces rejection. This enables you to feel even worse.

5

Preparing for Marriage Problems
(Poor Mate Selection)

This section is designed for those of you who hope to get married and are interested in developing marital problems. It will prove helpful to you even if you are married because you may get a divorce in the future. If you want problems, *start early*.

Marriage researchers suggest that the best way to build a good marriage is to begin with a wise choice for a mate. The obvious flip side would be that the best way to build a bad marriage is to begin with a poor choice for a mate. Such an obvious technique often is overlooked because we think we have no control over choosing the person with whom we "fall in love." This is a typical misconception of those people who have learned to excuse themselves from the responsibility of their own choices, who have learned to be the victims of their own emotions.

The truth is that we do have a lot of control over our choices. In fact, we usually *walk* into love. We seldom *fall* into it though we can certainly learn to fall *in* it. We can even apply some simple rules to be sure that we have problems built into our love relationships. A lot of people do this "unconsciously" already, so there is no reason for you not to do it consciously.

In the natural course of dating, you will meet a variety of people. You will then choose to continue dating one person. The question is, "How do you decide on that one person?" How do you find the courage to make a present choice when a worse selection may be waiting for you in the future? Of course, you cannot ever be absolutely sure you are choosing a loser, but the following rules may help you select a poor mate.

1. Select a poor communicator. Since effective communication is one of the most important functions in a healthy marriage, look for early signs of weakness in this area. If your dates talk all of the time, none of the time, or just don't seem to understand what you are trying to say, they deserve at least a second date. If there is difficulty in communicating during the dating time, you can be pretty sure it will get worse after marriage. All you have to do is apply the techniques taught in the following chapter to insure continuing difficulty.

2. Select someone with whom you have nothing in common. Look for someone who likes what you dislike; someone with whom you share no mutual interests. This is easier than you might guess. If you dislike music, hang around symphony halls, concerts, bandstands—anywhere you might meet music lovers. If you hate sports, take yourself out to the ball parks, ski resorts, sports and health clubs, tennis courts, stadiums, etc. You will find sports lovers there.

Once you find someone who likes what you dislike, you must pretend that you agree with him or her. Faking agreements requires more energy than being honest but it is worth it because it solidifies problems for the future.

When you pretend to like what your potential mate likes, you are developing a very powerful technique that can be used —and, indeed, is used—in marriage, as well as in hundreds of other areas of problem-development. My brother, Larry, taught me this very useful technique. We call it, "Lying in order to create trust." I sometimes call it pseudotrust.

My brother had a girl friend who was a singer. She asked him what he thought of her singing. He told her that he liked her singing, but she was not satisfied. She lied, "No, don't just say that. I want to know what you *really* think of my ability as a singer. Please feel free to be honest with me. I can take criticism, and I won't be upset at anything you say." She had created trust.

After a little coaxing and with some reluctance, he stated honestly, "Well, you have a nice voice, but I would suggest that you would be wise to look for a different profession. Sing for your own enjoyment."

She said, "Humph," and wouldn't speak to him for three weeks.

Lying to create trust is a technique used by anyone who says "I really want you to tell me what you think. I don't care if you criticize me." Anyone who says this convincingly can trick people into being honest. If you succeed in creating enough trust to elicit a critical comment, become angry, and your friend will be disillusioned and frustrated. You will have a problem.

It is wise not to reveal your hand during the dating time. Pretend that these honest criticisms do not bother you. At least keep up the pretense until after you are married. There will be plenty of time for anger after the exchange of vows.

3. Select someone who has fairly serious* hang-ups. One of the surest ways to have prolonged marital conflict is to marry someone who already has serious problems. Marry with the intention of helping, reforming or inspiring your prospective mate to become more than he or she is. You can seldom do any of those things, but they sound good. And certainly no one can blame *you* when future problems arise since you had such "good intentions." It is not only a way to insure your problems but also a way to avoid being blamed for them. Neat!

---

*Serious means serious to you. That can include any habit or characteristic that irritates you.

4. Select someone who is your opposite. This is a tricky and potentially sticky suggestion. Some people who marry opposites have very creative and satisfying relationships. They learn to blend their strengths, balance their relationships and allow one another enough freedom and space to grow as people.

The trick in marital problem-development is to find an opposite, with the intention of making that person become like you. After all, in marriage the two are supposed to become one. With that thought in the back of your mind, you can both begin to fight over which one of the two of you will be the one the two of you become! May the best, most right and strongest person win. You've got a problem!

5. Select on the basis of physical attraction alone. Follow your glands! Ignore common sense. Tell yourself that love (physical love) will conquer all.

We can be physically attracted to many people. And if physical attraction is the only bond holding a relationship together, the glow (and possibly the marriage) will be gone long before the first gray hairs, the first wrinkles or the first signs of flab appear to mar the physical perfection.

6. Select incompatible in-laws. Visit as much as possible with your prospective spouse's family. When you find a family with internal conflict, and most important, toward whom you feel personal hostility, then you have discovered real prospects for enduring conflict.

Tell yourself that it really doesn't matter because you are not going to marry the family anyway. Be as unrealistic as you can, and do nothing to overcome the tension. Let it smolder. If you are fortunate enough to marry into this family, you will have enough problems in reserve to last for years to come.

7. Select someone of whom you are unworthy. Of course, there are no such people, but, as in all areas of PROBLEM-PRODUCTION, facts mean nothing. You can select anyone and tell yourself you are not worthy of that person.

The mind set is important. Believe you are unworthy. Convince your potential mate that you are unworthy. This mind set gives you potential for two directions in the future:

a. You can keep yourself in a position of unworthiness that will eventually nauseate even the most patient mate. That person will become disgusted with an unworthy partner and probably leave you.

b. You can later resent your mate for believing he or she is better than you are. A real fight can grow from this germ.

There is a third possibility. You may be able to discard enough worthy mates until you finally find someone who is as unworthy—at least in comparison with the aforementioned worthies—as you believe yourself to be. You will then have a winning combination. The two of you can vie openly for the title of unworthiest.

8. Choose from two basic rules governing length of engagement:

a. Whomever you select, marry that person as soon as possible. The length of the engagement, however, is a function of how well you get to know your potential mate. The point is to marry before you have a chance to really get to know one another. That way you can avoid knowledge of flaws—such as angry creditors, active alcoholism, latent homosexuality or temporarily closeted exwives—which may cast shadows over what otherwise appeared to be a glowing and rosy future.

You certainly don't want impotency or frigidity to be the only surprise left for the marriage. The less you know, the more surprised you'll be. And besides the surprise, you have a nice safety valve for your own guilt when problems arise (and they will). You can always say, "Well, I had no idea that he/she was like that." That will be true—because you have seen to it.

b. Prolong the engagement beyond any reasonable expectation. This is a tactic of misogamists.* These are the ones who fake a desire to get married because of social or family pressures. They say they want to be married but will prolong engagements while waiting for guarantees. Guarantees never come, and neither does marriage. This is a fact the misogamist will pretend to bemoan into senescence.

9. Special suggestion for misopedists.**

If you really have trouble accepting or even liking children, the most positive possibility for problems in marriage is with a person who has children. Look for a person who has been married and has several children (no less than three).

You can resent any future time your spouse spends with those children, be jealous of any attention or money given to them, plan to participate as little as possible in their activities or their upbringing.

Summary: Review all of these suggestions before going on a date. Memorize them. Make them a part of your subconscious thought patterns, so that, even without thinking, you can make the right moves to assure poor mate selection. You are now ready to join the already married in reading the next chapter of this book, on the development of marital problems.

---

*According to *Mrs. Byrne's Dictionary of Unusual, Obscure and Preposterous Words* by Josepha Heifetz Byrne (The Citadel Press, Secaucus, New Jersey, 1974), *misogamy* is hatred of marriage.

**Misopedia*, according to Mrs. Byrne's Dictionary, is "hatred of children, especially your own."

6

Marriage Problems

Marriage relationships provide some of the most fertile fields for the growth of problems. In fact, most people need very little help here because in marriage you have the benefit of a partnership. Two heads *are* better than one.

In marriage you have not only your own problem-producing skills, but the cooperation of a partner who has similar but unique prejudices, limitations, preconceived notions, demands and, if you have chosen your mate wisely, a few irritating characteristics. It is my opinion that no marriage succeeds or fails through the efforts of one person alone, because either way it is a partnership.

I must hasten to add that you need not be discouraged if your partner doesn't want problems. If you learn and persistently apply the techniques described in this chapter, you can enlist your partner's cooperation in less than six days. (In the unlikely event that he or she refuses to get into PROBLEM-PRODUCTION, you can rest on the seventh day and begin the whole process of problem-creation again on the next day. Persist! Even Samson eventually gave in!)

If your marital problems thus far are just of the run-of-the-mill, nitpicking variety, and you'd like to escalate your level of expertise to qualify for at least a trial separation, take heed of the following suggestions. They will guarantee you at least one marital maladjustment to share with the world (or hopefully, with a well-qualified and hungry therapist).

Suggestion 1: Thwarting Communication

A discussion of communication has to come first because this is the most crucial area for all marital relationships. If you communicate honestly, openly, and often, you will have great difficulty generating serious problems. On the other hand, if you can learn to thwart communications, you will automatically be able to produce problems in almost every area of marital relationship.

Since communication tops the list and good communication seems vital to a well-functioning marriage, it stands to reason that bad communication would be vital to a poorly functioning marriage.

Most people seem to recognize the importance of communication. I have been conducting a little survey for myself. I have asked college students, church groups and counselees to list the three things they consider most important to a good marital relationship. The top vote-getter is communication. They also list love, respect, commitment, encouragement, mutual interests, cooperativeness and friendship high on their composite lists of needs for a happy marriage. But even though messing up *any* of these things will generate problems, it is clear that lousy communication will do it most efficiently and dramatically.

Begin with Mind Reading: Never take your mate's statements literally. Look for hidden meanings. Know what your mate is thinking even if nothing is actually said. Nothing frustrates a mate and thwarts his or her freedom to communicate more than a statement like, "Okay, I know what you said, but I also know what you really meant."

You can rave for hours at your defenseless mates if you keep telling them what they are thinking. No matter how much they deny, persist! Marriage can be pushed to the brink of destruction by a skillful mind reader. It doesn't matter that you may be wrong; in fact, the effect is even better when you *are* wrong.

The possibilities are endless. "You don't like (this or that) ..." "You didn't have a good time at ..." "You were uncomfortable because ..." "You don't really want to ..." This is mind reading!

The logical complement to your own mind-reading act is the insistence that your mate develop the same skill. Never tell your spouse what you think or want. Expect him or her to know. Say, "If you really cared (or loved me), you would know." There is no defense from that attack. It will produce frustrations which lead to lingering marital conflict.

Learn to Overreact: Exaggerate your normal reactions, because this simple tactic tips a relationship out of balance immediately. Throw a temper tantrum over some insignificant mishap. If you can do it publicly, the results will be both intense and fast.

I worked with one couple who had a two-month fight over a biscuit. One biscuit was left on the platter, and dinner was nearly finished. She placed the biscuit on his plate, and he artistically overreacted. "What the hell do you think I am? A garbage disposal?" With just a few more well-chosen remarks, there developed what I now refer to as "the great biscuit controversy."

I'm sure most psychologists would say this overreaction was symptomatic of a deeper problem. This may have been the case in this particular situation, but you do not have to have deeper problems. You can overreact to almost anything, real or imagined. Use overstatement or overreaction to *start* a problem.

Create Defensiveness: If you can communicate in such a way that you make your mate feel challenged, criticized, judged or condemned, you can stimulate defensiveness. This will move the focus away from understanding and/or solving a problem to one of self-defense and/or counter-attack. This process is so simple that even newlyweds can do it.

The first step is to avoid taking responsibility for anything. Never admit that you are wrong regardless of the circumstances. It is a short step from ducking responsibility to producing defensiveness. This step is taken by blaming or accusing your mate. "It's your fault." It makes no difference how ridiculous or irrational the accusation is. It still works.

Confuse Issues: You can easily generate a problem in communication by not permitting a topic to be discussed reasonably. Blur the focus by bringing in irrelevant issues. For example, let us say the topic is making decisions without consulting your mate. At the first break in the conversation, actively insert ambiguity with a statement such as, "Well, I really don't see why you're so steamed up, and besides that, your mother has caused trouble between us since the first day we were married, and you are careless with money."

Use Irritating Phrases: I had one client who drove her spouse to distraction by saying, "But that's not the point." No matter what they discussed, no matter what he said, she always chimed in, "But that's not the point." Some other irritating phrases include: "So what?" or "That's just the way I am;" "You should have thought of that before you got married;" "You never ..." or "You always ..." And, if all else fails, the standard "I told you so" will be irritating enough to create problems.

Use Passive Communication: Passive communication is talk with no action. Effective communication, like good golf, requires follow-through.

Talk without action is like faith without works. It is dead. It becomes deader with each passive conversation and soon produces a condition I call *spouse deafness*. Say things you have no intention of doing, such as, "The next time you don't pick up your clothes, I'm going to burn them or the house," or, "The next time you are late, I'm going to kill you or your mother or both." Modify these statements to fit your own circumstances.

The genuine passive communicators use all their steam to blow their whistles. They never have any power left to produce action. If you are successful at passive communication, your mate will become so spouse deaf that he or she will be able to read a good book (or any book) comfortably while you scream obscenities and threats.

When this condition is fully developed, you will feel totally discounted and blame your spouse for your frustration. Like all good problem-producing techniques, passive communication is woven into the warp and woof of the total marriage relationship.

Use Silence: As a last resort, you can give your partner "The Silent Treatment." Refuse to discuss the matter (whatever it is that needs discussing). The record for the silent treatment, so far as I know, is nine weeks, three days, two hours and twelve minutes.* One woman came to me for help after her husband had stopped talking to her when she refused to fix an evening meal. He had not spoken to her for more than eight weeks, and she was in a terrible emotional state.

I was trying to devise a therapeutic intervention for her when help came from an unexpected source. Their silent siege was aborted when his mother made a surprise visit to their home. Beginners in the use of silence often permit themselves to be thwarted by intrusions from visitors. With practice, the

---

*The minutes are approximations because it was hard to know exactly when the silence began.

silent antagonists can keep the veil drawn, even in the presence of guests, by talking around each other.

Well-adjusted couples seem to talk openly and honestly about their relationships. If you want problems—stop talking!

Suggestion 2: Screwing Up Sex

Another easy area in which you can produce problems is that of the sex relationship or the erotic zone. When people are giving themselves in this most intimate relationship, their feelings are as bare and vulnerable as their bodies.

Before beginning to work on your feelings about sex, it is appropriate to point out that sex problems have their beginnings *in our attitudes*—rotten attitudes generate rotten situations.

You may have picked up your basic rotten attitudes from parents, friends, "education," or through religious "training."

If you are among the more fortunate people, you were brought up by a mother or father who referred to your exploration of genitals (either yours or those of a friend or sibling) as "Playing Nasty." As in, "Now don't you Play Nasty." (When I first heard that, I thought it meant I should wash my genitals thoroughly before proceeding. I quickly learned what Mom really meant when she said nasty.*)

Think of sex as dirty: The standard, and still one of the most useful, poor attitudes is that sex is dirty or bad. Even if you do not really believe sex is dirty or bad, you still can get some of the same negative results by pretending. Anytime your partner wishes to discuss sex or to improve the sexual relationship, respond by saying, "That's disgusting." Or, "That

---

Nasty, according to Mrs. Byrne's Dictionary, is the same as *immund*, which is an adjective meaning "filthy, dirty; filthy dirty."

nauseates me." Or, "Don't be silly, I can't talk about that." Even if these statements are not true, they will generate negative attitudes in your partner.

One couple with tremendous potential for sex problems abruptly halted their premarital counseling sessions with me after I had inadvertently referred to his genital organ as a penis. What I actually said was, "The fact that he has a penis, and you don't, doesn't mean that you cannot relate as equals."

They never returned to my office but her mother called me with the explanation. "They are not coming back to see you, because they were shocked that a clergyman would use such language."

In my innocence I asked, "What language?"

She said, "Well, you said ..." Then she whispered into the telephone mouthpiece, "Penis."

"Oh," I replied, as if I understood. "What do they call it?"

I never found the answer to my question, but I fantasized that they will refer to it as "his thing" as they generate their sexual conflicts.

Think of sex as duty: Cultural influence has made this specifically useful to the female, though not exclusively so. When you can think of sex in terms of duty,* you reduce the possibility that you will enjoy it. "Well, if you must, go ahead. I want to be a good wife, and this is part of what I see as my responsibility." Husbands can aid in the development of this attitude by accusing their wives of feeling that way, whether they do or not. "You are a lousy wife. You don't even live up to *your* obligations in the bedroom."

It is important to remember that in the bedroom as well as in most other areas of marital conflict, truth is not necessary. Problems can be generated just as effectively and at times more effectively by false accusations or by commitment to a

---

*The more proficient producers of sexual problems think sex is dirty duty.

myth. Many people are mythomaniacs* anyway, so ignore truth.

Do not ask for specific behavior from your spouse: Clarifying your sexual desires is a sure way to avoid sexual problems. Problem-producers are never open with their mates about sexual feelings and wants.

One couple with a lot of sexual conflict came to me for counseling. After four sessions she told me that his foreplay really "turned her off."

He was shocked! "I can't believe that. Why, every time I rub your stomach you become so excited you can't be still."

She looked at the floor and blushed.

"Is that true?" I asked.

Very meekly and still clearly embarrassed she confessed, "I move because it tickles me."

Imagine that! For almost seven years he was touching her with the belief that he was exciting her when in fact he was tickling her!

He never asked and she never told. You can apply this silence about sex to anything your spouse fails to do that you would like or that your spouse is doing that you do not like. You will maintain your present problems and continue to develop new ones.

Think of sex as a reward or punishment: This is the thinking that precedes a maneuver which enables either spouse to withhold the sexual expression of love until the other has done something "deserving" of such expressions.

The flip side of this problem-producing attitude is the idea that withholding sex is a punishment for a spouse's failure to behave properly.

Of course, you don't have to say these things openly. They are much more effective if used in subtle, but clear, ways. If

---

*According to Mrs. B's Dictionary, *mythomania* is compulsively telling lies and believing them.

the message is not getting through to your partner, you can always opt to be more specific.

For example: "Did you ever fix that drain spout on the back of the house?"

"Yes, I repaired it this morning and even painted it to cover the dents."

"Great. Let's go to bed."

Or you may use the opposite approach.

"Did you call the plumber today like I asked you?"

"Oh, no! I forgot."

"Well, you go on to bed. I think *I'll* sit up for about four or five hours."

Once you get reward and punishment built into your sexual relationship, you'll have bedroom problems for years.

Believe that sex is for men only: This concept is becoming more and more difficult to use, but an amazingly large number of people manage to keep it alive. The idea is to convince yourselves that men need sex in order to survive. Feed yourselves the myth that the man's drive is stronger. "If he doesn't have sex, the semen will build up and create excruciating pain!" Never mind celibates, or the fact that men seem to survive even without sex. I've heard of some men living alone on desert islands for as long as one hour without sex! Say to yourselves, "After all, a really good woman doesn't actually enjoy sex—certainly not very much." (In marriages where this is believed it is usually true.)

One couple I met had believed these myths for years, and their sexual problems became chronic when the wife actually initiated sex one night. She dared to hint that she really wanted "it."

This skilled problem-producing husband said, "I couldn't believe it. I never heard anyone but a prostitute speak that way." (I wonder how he knew that!)

Believe in doubt: Communicate doubt to your spouse by doubting him or her. Absolutely refuse to believe any positive statement made by your mate, especially if that statement concerns sex.

State plainly, "I do not believe you really had an orgasm. You are only saying that because you are afraid I'll be hurt if you didn't. You don't really enjoy sex with me. You are faking."

A modification of the Pyrite Rule applies in the area of doubt: If you doubt others, they will doubt you. Doubt your mate's sexual communication, and your mate will doubt your sexual communication. Once this state of suspicion has been established, the vulnerable and exposed feelings of both you and your spouse can be injured regularly.

Expect perfect sexual response: Tell yourself that if you have a true love relationship, your spouse will want sex every time you do and vice versa. Tell yourself that if yours is the right kind of marriage, you and your spouse will almost always experience simultaneous orgasm. But *certainly*, regardless of circumstances, when one does, both will. These expectations will never be consistently realized, and even when they are fulfilled, you should be able to doubt that you are being told the truth.

Insure failure with poor timing. A perfect time to snuggle up to your mate and ask whether sex is the top priority on his or her agenda is when your partner is suffering one of those viruses characterized by a slight fever of two or three degrees, nausea, and a general feeling of malaise. I need not point out to you the obvious disappointment you can experience through the rejection you will read into this circumstance. On the other hand, if you are the diseased party, acquiesce with great dignity, so that you can feel martyred and used ("only a body ... no concern for my well-being") for literally months to come.

Reduce foreplay to a minimum:* Rush! Why wait when *you*

---

*Forty-five seconds, at the most.

are ready now? Leave the foreplay to those who are skilled at intimacy. They are not good problem-producers. Problem-producers forego foreplay. I could say more about this, but I want to hurry on.

Remember that crude remarks are a turn-off: You can always negatively affect your partner's attitude through using ammunition from your armory of carefully selected crude remarks. One problem-producing couple with whom I have worked has scaled the zenith in the compilation of cutting, crude remarks.

She says to him, "You are about as skilled in lovemaking as a dog with brain damage." She snarlingly adds, "You must be among the top five clumsiest lovers in the world." These remarks are indelibly engraved in their scrapbook of bedroom memories when she laughs at his attempts to initiate sex.

He retaliates with, "You are just a frigid cake of ice in the bed. It would take an acetylene torch to warm you up." He now has reduced foreplay to, "Let's hit the sheets, Icey."

I heard of one man who apoligizes to his wife during sex by saying, "Oh, I'm sorry. I must have hurt you because I felt you move." A wife sets her husband up for trouble by beginning their sexual encounters with, "Would you wake me up when you're finished, I have some reading to do."

Inappropriate remarks or actions deepen the hurt in sexual partners. During intense foreplay either partner can abruptly change the atmosphere by saying something like, "Oh, that reminds me, did you pay the gas bill?"

One of the most clever ideas for producing sexual problems was reported to me by a World War II veteran who served in the Philippines and once cohabited with a prostitute who ate oranges during their tender encounter. (Crackers or cookies make good substitutes here.)

Pick a fight at night: It is extremely helpful in problem-generation to "pick a fight" at bedtime and then go to bed without resolving the problem. Without further comment or apology, move directly into sexual foreplay, a technique guaranteed to confuse your partner and create a lingering hostility. This is not especially creative, but it is a quickie that is effective.

Use mind reading and self-talk: Mind reading is useful in sexual conflict production. One example of this comes from a man who always read his wife's meaning beyond her words. He would lie down beside her with thoughts of sexual activity on his mind; then the following conversation would take place. (The parenthetical expressions are his thoughts and may or may not have anything to do with reality.)

He: "How are you feeling tonight?"

She: "I'm really tired. How about you?"

He: (That means she doesn't want to have sex with me tonight. Rejected again! Crap!) "Oh, I'm fine." Then skillfully hooking the cover over his left shoulder he abruptly turns away from her.

She: "What's wrong?"

He: (If she had any sensitivity at all, she'd know—but she doesn't care that much.) Angrily, "Nothing. Why?"

She: "You seem bothered!"

He: (Bothered, hell! There's one for the books. She rejects me, pretends not to know what bothers me then says, "You seem bothered.") Innocently, "I can't understand that. Go on to sleep."

After fifteen to twenty minutes of restless turning and self-talk including silent remarks to himself like, "I don't see how she can possibly sleep knowing how upset I am," he throws the covers back and gets up with a blast, "Well, there's no point in my trying to sleep *now*." The fight is on.

Once you start combining mind reading and self-talk, the possibilities are endless. A creative person can use this technique to generate a lifetime of problems.

Read rotten material: What you read is important but what not to read is also very important. There is plenty of "trash" available. You can confuse yourself by reading as many "adult" stories as possible. When you get your sex drive untracked, it will probably become totally insatiable. Expectations drawn from much of the literature and movie material today can be raised (or lowered) to the point that you will always be frustrated.

If you want problems, stay away from factual materials on sex. Do not read any of the reputably researched materials available in sex manuals. Feast your mind on "kinky" materials. You can exasperate your spouse by insisting on having sex only as you swing from the chandelier, swim underwater (wearing snorkel equipment), hang from a parachute while your neighbors look on (or join in).

Never share tenderness without intercourse: Every happily married couple I have known shared times of warmth, caressing, kissing and hugging, even when they are not planning to have intercourse.

To insure sexual problems, insist on sexual intercourse every time you express any physical love. I assure you that persisting in this pattern will reward you with future comments such as, "You only touch me when you want sex."

Conclusion: Once you have mastered these easy techniques for producing sexual problems, you can guarantee continuing sexual misery by absolutely refusing to discuss any of the embryonic or fully developed sexual conflicts you have parented in your bedroom.

Suggestion 3: Creative Jealousy

Marriage involves two people's commitment to join in the mutual task of living together. But in order to develop jealousy, a major problem in marriage, you must discard that apparently mundane concept and develop, instead, the concept of ownership.

Developing the concept of ownership is the first and most important step toward jealousy in marriage. Create in yourself the image that title to a new piece of property is being transferred to you when the wedding bands are exchanged. Something like being handed the keys and title to a new car.

Claim exclusive rights: Say to yourself, "I have exclusive rights to my wife/husband. I have the right to demand his or her total attention." This will help you to feel threatened even if your spouse merely talks to a member of the opposite sex, when your spouse spends time or money on his or her children,* when your spouse does anything without your clinging presence.

Use your imagination: The development of imagination, too often abandoned in childhood, is a tremendous asset in developing jealousy. I know one man who can construct such a vivid picture of imagined infidelity involving his wife and numerous other men that he remains in a constant state of misery. His ensuing jealousy makes life miserable for his wife as well. He even makes their friends (the few friends they have) uncomfortable with his innuendos. He often makes open accusations, which although usually directed at his wife, are intended for the benefit of anyone who may hear.

Try it the next time you drive away from your spouse. Begin by imagining that the phantom lover has learned your schedule or that your spouse called that lover while your goodby kisses were still lingering on the lips. Think of all the things they might be saying to one another. Soon you'll almost be able to hear them laughing. Stop reading this second. Dial your spouse, very slowly, making sure you hit the correct

---

*The children may be yours or belong to your spouse from a previous marriage.

digits. If you get a busy signal, or fail to get an answer, you don't need me to tell you what you are now imagining.

Build mountains: This is the process through which small, relatively insignificant incidents heap up until they are full-fledged controversies.

If you've never built mountains, you'll find what I'm about to tell you hard to believe, but it actually happened. A man saw his wife shake hands with another man at a church event. Imagine that! They actually touched! That's all he needed. In his mind they were holding hands, and no one does that unless they're having an affair. From a hand shake to the bedroom! That is real mountain building. It was so effective that when I saw them and heard the problem told with vigor and anger, I could hardly conceal my disbelief. Not only had it been a major controversy in the family for more than twenty years, but it was one of the catalysts that led to their ultimate divorce. Although you may not be able to build such a great mountain from such a small molehill, you can certainly learn to build adequate mountains.

Conclusion: Remember that suspicion and doubt are essential to the generation of jealousy. I learned a very simple rule from one of my counselees, which will help you keep your mind moving toward bigger and better jealousy. Apply it when your spouse is late. Or when you are alone and wondering what your spouse is doing in your absence. The rule is: "When in doubt, doubt."

Suggestion 4:
Making a Problem Out of Problem-Solving

Problem-solving has been receiving a lot of attention from those in the helping professions who are interested in seeing couples build better marriages. Some contend that all marriages have at least a few problem areas, so they try to teach couples the art of problem-solving. This is an ideal place to do PROBLEM-PRODUCTION. If you can make a problem out of problem-solving, you are assured of some long-term marital conflict.

Timing is one key to making a mess out of the problem-solving process. The more inconvenient the time, the more likely you are to derail any honest attempts by your partner to problem-solve. Pick the worst possible time, or even an impossible time, to discuss your problems.

One neat trick is to bring up an issue which has made you angry when your mate doesn't have time to respond. Say you both are going to a wedding, and your spouse is slow in getting ready. You know you're going to be late, and you are irritated. Just as you arrive, ten minutes late, give your mate a real verbal blast and leap out of the car without allowing time for a response. Name-calling will further complicate the situation. A good parting shot might be, "You are so damn slow it is stupid. We always arrive late, and thanks to your insensitivity, it's always your fault. You've got to be the slowest person in the world with the possible exception of your mother."

Dragging in mother-in-law is a stroke of genius. To cap off this trick, do not wait for a response, get out, slam the door and begin your brisk walk to your destination. (Be sure you have the only keys to the car or else a ride home!)

Another good time to bring up problems is just when your mate is leaving the house for work. It will be more effective if you select a morning when your spouse has overslept. Wait until he or she is rushing out the door. If by chance your mate decides to be late for work and offers to talk then you can make a strategic retreat to the bathroom.

My favorite poor-timing suggestion is "the 3 a.m. eye-opener." Nothing handicaps the would-be problem solver more than to be awakened with an angry shake at three in the morning. While he or she is still groggy, rapidly spell out in detail your complaint. By the time your spouse is fully awake you'll have a good fight going.

Overload the conversation. If you do get trapped into a problem-solving session with your mate, there are several effective maneuvers sure to prevent any real progress. Overloading is one of these effective techniques. This is the process by which you gradually add more and more issues to the discussion. (You may wish to refine overloading through referring back to "Snowballing" and "Confusing the Issue.") Never wait for one problem to be resolved; just keep adding to it.

If your present complaint is that your spouse leaves the cap off the toothpaste tube, wait until some progress is being made toward a solution; then add, "Well, besides that, you always give me the cold shoulder when I want to have sex, and you never have enough time to talk to me." Later you can add, "We always go where you want to go, and your family never has liked me."

Overloading is easy and effective. Remember, specificity is the enemy of PROBLEM-PRODUCTION.

Be mulish. This is a Missouri term for insisting on your own way or being stubborn. Make up your mind from the beginning that your way of handling the situation or resolving the problem is the only acceptable one. Take a non-negotiable stand. Refuse to compromise. Say to yourself that compromise is defeat and you won't stand for it.

The idea that defeat and victory are the only possible alternatives leads to a non-compromising and strongly competitive position. Once the concept of "must win" is grounded in both partners, the relationship will lose.

The happiest couples I know have learned the art of compromising. If you refuse to accept compromise on any issue, you are assured of real problems.

Sidetracking* the discussion. This is different from overloading, though the effect on your partner is similar. If you can make your spouse angry enough to forget the issue, you are assured of no progress. One of the simplest techniques for sidetracking is name-calling. Experiment until you discover what names irritate the most and use them with great emphasis at the outset of each agrument.

For example, call your mate stupid, a female canine, or an ignorant man still searching for his father. Name calling will generate defensiveness and sidetrack most discussions. This is a good way to be sure the discussion goes nowhere—and goes there for a long time.

Blaming or faulting is an equally effective tool. Forget the issue and fight about who is responsible. You can spend all of your available time in accusations and counteraccusations. Most people are more skilled at debating who is to blame than they are at solving problems, so it is not difficult to pull the average mate into such a debate. All you have to say is, "It's all your fault anyway" and you are again sidetracked.

Leave it up in the air. Avoid at all cost a specific solution to your problems. Later when you fail to follow through, you can say, "Oh, I never understood it that way." You are then ready to start the whole process over again.

Suggestion 5: Stunting Growth

If you wake up some morning and discover that growth has occurred in your marital relationship or if your partner seems to be maturing and changing gracefully, you can easily put a stop to that process.

---

*Sidetracking is an old railroad term. It means that cars are taken off the main track. Side tracks seldom lead anywhere.

Everyone probably knows that growth or change takes place in an accepting, tolerant, supportive and encouraging atmosphere. Because growth is enhanced by positive comments and compliments, I often suggest a series of exercises to couples with whom I am working. I ask each of the to spend a little time everyday focusing on warm and good experiences* shared with his/her spouse in the past. Try, I ask them, to substitute this for reminding each other of the bad times. I have even suggested that couples consciously try to say and do positive and supportive things for one another at least once every day. I ask each spouse to keep a record, without consulting the other, of the positive things they do and say. Each keeps a second list for the positive things they have observed the spouse doing for them or saying to them. Then at the next session, we share the results of all this conscious attempt to appreciate and encourage.

If your relationship is good and growing, you do not need the specific exercise mentioned above. What you need are some ideas for stunting the growth you have been experiencing. This is such a simple process that I'm amazed when people haven't discovered it for themselves. Simply stated, you just reverse the atmosphere of growth. Substitute rejection for acceptance, intolerance for tolerance, competition for support and criticism for encouragement.

Always criticize: Perhaps the most powerful block to growth is constant criticism. (This is effective with children, too.) No one feels free to change in the hostile atmosphere of criticism. Be picky, nag, complain, find areas to criticize. Never compliment your mate, and if you ever slip and do so, make sure you offset the error with at least six criticisms.

One woman said to me, concerning the power of criticism, "I should have known how it affected him (her husband) because

---

*I sometimes suggest that both people independently think of a couple of experiences from their past together which were especially pleasant. They then share them with each other. This is often the first time they've focused on good times in a long time.

of how it affects me. I get angry when I am criticized, and I never feel like doing better when that happens." Think about it. If you really want to stunt growth in your partner, think of the things that hinder your growth and do those things to him or her. One far wiser than I said, "Do unto others as you would have them do unto you." Just reverse that principle if you want to stunt growth. Stated in terms of PROBLEM-PRODUCTION it would read, "Do unto others what would bother you if they did it unto you."

Freeze the status quo: This is another way of saying, "Kill your relationship." Only dead things do not grow or change. One never-fail method for producing an atmosphere of discouragement is to laugh at the attempts your mate makes at change.

Smirk: "If you could see yourself now, you'd just die! You look so silly."

Giggle: "You're beginning to sound like one of those kooky personal-growth nuts."

Soon even the most determined person will stop trying. Discouragement generated by laughing criticism is devastating. (Note: Anytime you can combine two or more techniques, the effect is magnified.)

Bear in mind that what you do to another, you can do to yourself through self-talk. Tell yourself that you look or sound foolish. Or preferably both. Remember that what you say does not have to be true or rational. Believe it, practice it, and it becomes true for you.

Always reject people who challenge you to grow: Reject anyone, but especially spurn would-be catalysts to growth. Refuse to talk to them. Refuse to look at them. Take advantage of any opportunity to walk away. This behavior achieves two things:

a. It helps you to avoid contact with growth-producing people. This immediately reduces the threat that you might grow.

b. When your spouse observes your deliberate rejection of other people who are growing, he or she will certainly be less likely to risk change.

Conclusion: To discourage growth, make use of criticism, holding the status quo and rejection. Underscore the whole process by adopting a motto like "Change is frightening, and growing is for children."

Suggestion 6: Double that Bind

Another useful technique in developing marital problems is putting your mate in a double bind—a "damned if you do and damned if you don't" situation.

Demand mutually exclusive proofs of love: One husband came home on a Thursday evening and said to his wife (who also worked outside the home) that he was going on a week-end trip, and if she loved him she'd wash and iron some shirts for him to take along. Then he nonchalantly added that he wouldn't be able to help her because this was his bowling night. And away he went. He returned home clad in his basset hound syndrome and dragging his bowling bag. His explanation was that he was the only one on his bowling team whose wife wasn't there to cheer him on. The very next time he wants proof of love, she will be in the double bind.

The wife is caught. If she had left the ironing and gone with him, what do you suppose? That's right! He would have complained that if she really loved him, she would have stayed home and done the washing and ironing. She was in a double bind, and she'll feel it coming the very next time he demands proof of love. This is good for producing months of fighting over whether or not one is loved—or almost anything else.

How about this one, wives? Announce to your husband that

you are now going to become a totally independent person. Demand, however, that he provide you with sufficient financial and affectional security to assure you of total independence. It is obviously impossible to be totally independent while relying on anyone else to provide financial and affectional security.

Accuse your mate of never permitting you to make the first move in sexual relations and then complain that he *never* approaches you. The list of double binds is nearly endless. Make up some for yourself. You can do it.

A second way to impose a double bind on your mate is to send dual messages. This is a sure-fire problem-producer. It is absolutely foolproof. Examples are so numerous it was hard for me to select only a couple.

For one example, try telling your mate that you want him or her to decide how to spend the evening. Ask, "What would you *really* like to do?" After learning what he or she would like, you can complain, "You *always* do what *you* want to do." (Save this complaint until you have arrived at the place your mate selected or even after you return home.) After a few experiences of this kind, your mate will stop believing you. That is perfect. You can now make this accusation: "You never believe anything I say."

Another example: One couple I know has had some wonderful fights because "she never listens to me." When she listens, he says, "She never talks to me." This is like telling your spouse to kick you, then later saying, "You'll be sorry you did that." When you really want to fight, you don't need a reason —you can make one up. The Double Bind is always a good starter. No person or relationship can remain comfortable while sitting on the horns of a dilemma.

Suggestion 7: Expect the Impossible

In my research and in my observations of counselees, I have discovered that the major cause for marital unhappiness is the gap that exists between expectation and fulfillment. It would follow that a sure and quick way to increase marital misery is to broaden the gap between hope and reality. In order to achieve this, all we have to do is promote a lot of myths about marriage.

The more unrealistic and impossible your expectations, the more confident you can be that you will always be disappointed. A few suggestions should get any of you started toward impossible goals and assure you of disappointment in your marriage.

It will be enough to simply list these suggestions. They speak for themselves. If you want to fail in marriage, or at least create an unhappy relationship, go into marriage with the following expectations and hang on to them no matter how irrational they are:

Expect your spouse always to understand your feelings and moods. No matter what time of day or night, no matter what his or her own feeling or mood, no matter what his or her physical condition, tell yourself, "If my spouse loved me he or she would surely understand." *No one* can live up to this expectation.

Expect that every time you want sex, your mate should want sex. Again, do not take into consideration personal differences, timing, physical condition, etc. Just expect your companion to always be ready. It helps if you also expect your partner to be understanding when you do not feel like responding to his or her desires. A satyric married to a nymphomaniac stands a chance.

Expect that you will never again feel lonely or unloved now that you are married. Demand constant companionship and a supportive relationship in every way. No matter what you do, expect to *feel* loved.

Expect your spouse to like everything you like, like every person you like and enjoy all the same activities you enjoy. "After all," you can say to yourself, "we ought to be able to share *everything.*"

Expect that neither your spouse nor your relationship will ever change in any way. Everything will remain as it was on the day you were married, and any deviation in pattern or person will be met negatively with, "But that's not the way we've always been. I'm afraid you don't love me like you used to."

The simple fact is that if you expect the impossible and refuse to alter your expectations, you will be assured of ultimate disappointment with your marriage. This gives you grounds for complaining about things that your partner will find humanly impossible to achieve. You now have your insurance that problems will always exist in your marriage.

Unrealistic expectations can and should be applied to all areas of marriage. It is the paste that holds the whole strategy for marital conflict together. I sum it up appropriately with a paraphrase from the nuptial vows. "Expect the impossible from marriage and ye shall be together till conflict and disillusionment do ye part."

7

Walling the Generation Gap

In PROBLEM-PRODUCTION we do not *bridge* the generation gap. We wall it or we broaden it! It is not a difficult task because children and young people are naturally suspicious of adults anyway. With just a little effort we can confirm the fact that we are against them. Following are tried and proven techniques for insuring rotten relationships with children.

Keep them quiet: One thing that keeps children off balance is never to allow them a voice in any of the decisions that involve them. Any time your children voice opinions, tell them they are "to be seen, not heard." This approach almost always leaves the pathetic little creature feeling "put down" and alienated. Children are easily discouraged anyway, and therefore by never permitting them to share in the decision-making process, we not only make them suspicious of us, we also begin to tear down their self-concepts. This assures them of problems in the future.

Attack, attack: With children, as on many battle fronts, the best defense is a good offense. If you can find any reason to attack or criticize your children, they will become defensive. This will keep them from regarding you as an ally. When parents consistently attack and criticize children, their suspicion and prediction that the younger generation does not trust older people will be confirmed.

Through the use of silencing and attacking children, adults aid in the establishment of devastating mutual distrust.

Ridicule: I suggest that you take advantage of every opportunity to ridicule children, especially in front of their friends. You can thus fill them with enough resentment to last for several weeks and assure you of their eventual retaliation. It is vital to keep ridiculing as much as possible, especially with younger children. They have an uncanny ability to forgive and forget unless there is *overwhelming* evidence that you are against them.

Set impossible goals for them: If you have a *small* son who is interested in intellectual pursuits, push him to become a football fullback or lineman. Tell him how important it is to you for him to make the varsity team. You can be sure that you will soon give him enough evidence of his failure to create confusion within him for years to come. In addition, you'll give him a head start on PROBLEM-PRODUCTION, because he will have a built-in failure expectation and can be expected to go through life trying to reach unreasonable goals.

If the stork delivers you a child with "average" intellectual ability, you can push him or her to excel in all studies. Set an educational goal of graduating with honors from high school — then of earning a B.A., an M.S. or M.A., followed by a Ph.D. and maybe an M.D. This will build up a lot of resentment toward you and will make communications shaky at best.

Scream the impossible scream: Yelling at children produces fear and defensiveness in them, but if you yell *impossible* threats at them, they will soon stop fearing you—and then stop listening to you. Threaten things you have neither the intention nor the means for doing. Even the slowest child will soon learn that you do not mean what you say. I use this easy-to-remember formula to help me break down communication with my children: 1) Talk, 2) Do Not Act, and, 3) When in Doubt, YELL.

Examples of the impossible screams* are:

"IF YOU DON'T STOP INTERRUPTING, I WILL KILL YOU."

"IF YOU DON'T PAY ATTENTION TO ME, YOU WILL NEVER BE PERMITTED OUT OF THIS HOUSE AGAIN."

"IF YOU DON'T EAT EVERYTHING ON YOUR PLATE, I'M GOING TO SEND ALL YOUR FOOD TO INDIA (OR CHINA, OR AFRICA) AND YOU WILL NEVER GET ANOTHER BITE OF FOOD IN THIS HOUSE AGAIN." (The danger with this statement is that a child who believes you might burn the house down).

"IF I EVER HEAR YOU USE THAT KIND OF LANGUAGE AGAIN, I WON'T SPEAK TO YOU AGAIN UNTIL HELL FREEZES OVER." (Promises, promises.)

Never be satisfied: A friend told me of one father, watching from poolside, who was called to the low diving board by his little boy, who excitedly wanted to demonstrate his ability to dive. He made his big splash and climbed out of the swimming pool, grinning proudly. His father, an expert in generating problems with and for children, disinterestedly said, "That was fine, son. Now when are you going off the high board?" His son, with much more training like that, will become frustrated with his father and never be satisfied with himself. There will always be a "higher board" for him in life.

The insatiable expectations of parents like those described above will destroy whatever good could be done with expres-

*All these statements should be made in a much louder than normal voice.

sions of appreciation for what Behavior Modification people call "small approximations," which are achievements somewhat short of ultimate goals or far short of perfection. For instance, riding a tricycle is a small approximation of riding a bicycle. Those of you learning PROBLEM-PRODUCTION should never permit a child to be satisfied with an approximation of future goals. Be satisfied with nothing short of perfection. This assures you of never being satisfied with the accomplishments of your child, while making it difficult for the child to be satisfied with any of his or her own achievements.

Parents frequently achieve the same level of discouragement for their children by doing things over for them. For example, if your child draws a picture for you, correct the picture, redraw the outlines, shade in all the proper places. This is guaranteed to discourage the child.

Wield your power: Remember that as long as you have some kind of power over your children, you can force them (reluctantly, of course) to do your bidding. Your power rests initially with your superior size. You can force them physically, through any number of barbarian approaches, to do what you want them to do—until they reach adolescence. Your power then evolves into manipulation with material items, such as clothes, money, cars, etc. Parents who have effectively developed the power approach say things like, "As long as you drive *my* car, eat *my* food and live under *my* roof, you'll do as I say."

When your child grows beyond these powers, you will clearly see the "generation gap," because as you lose power to *force* obedience, you will have no more control and very little influence.

The effective use of power, and refusal to use reason or to use any democratic approaches in family discussions, will not only destroy the child's respect for you, but will create resentment for all authority. Then your children may some day become full-blown rebels, and you'll have the problem you've been anticipating.

Avoid all forms of encouragement: Avoid communicating acceptance and understanding. People respond so positively to this dynamic duo that you can ruin a whole year's PROBLEM-PRODUCTION by merely communicating such encouragements.

It is also important to avoid *any* encouraging remarks in order to produce truly discouraged offspring. The troubled home is a home where "never is heard an encouraging word."

Flaunt the good old days: You can ice over your poor relationship by constantly making references to the superior behavior of kids, including yourself, when you were a child. If you need a clincher, you can always throw in the "good old days." This will certainly keep the "bad days" rolling along in your family.

Remember that families who function well together are characterized by the time they spend talking with each other, by their use of compromise in dealing with problems, by an absence of physical, psychological, and material force, and by the presence of encouragement.

Save them from consequences: If you want to create a good foundation for fostering future delinquency, never permit your children to experience natural or logical consequences of their behavior. If they oversleep, do not permit them to be late for school or to be inconvenienced in any way by their own behavior. Drive them there, if necessary. Or if all else fails, write them an excuse. Teach them that no matter what they do, you will protect them from any negative consequences.

When you are able to protect children sufficiently from inconvenience, work and the responsibility for their own behavior, you help them to become spoiled tyrants.

Such children become unemployed adults because all the jobs for tyrants, princes and princesses have been filled. There are not even many openings for frogs.

My oldest son, who is almost 16, borrowed and later broke a friend's watch. With rare and great restraint I did not offer to replace the watch. Though it was painful for me, I permitted him to use his savings, plus a loan of three dollars against his next week's allowance, to buy a new watch for his friend.

I said, "Bill, I'm sorry to see you having to spend your money for a watch." (He was starting a savings account for his first car.)

He dejectedly replied, "That's all right, Dad. I'll get over it in a few weeks. And besides, we have to suffer the logical consequences of our behavior."

Evidently I have not helped him develop as much problem-producing behavior as I might have.

My personal belief is that parents, through their laziness, selfishness and guilt help children produce problems—by spoiling them, not permitting them to experience the consequences of their own behavior, and by failing to spend time talking with or listening to them.

Special note to teachers: You will soon discover that many parents do not want you to teach their children anything. They do not want their children to be challenged too much by being assigned homework. They want only to hear your good comments concerning their children.

A good many administrators do not want trouble with parents, so they, too, will often dislike any teacher who makes waves by expecting students to learn.

Make your professional contributions to the world of PROBLEM-PRODUCTION by not expecting your students to grow in the development of educational skills. Become a glorified babysitter.

Never permit students to have fun while they are learning, and never force them to do anything they don't have fun doing. In this way you will assure yourself of remaining in the good graces of parents and administrators, as well as making certain that you have done nothing to improve your students' futures.

8

Free-floating Problems: Anxiety and Worry

Anxiety and worry are probably best explained and understood as fears we learn to feel. Fear becomes neurotic when it becomes unreasonable. One of the beauties about PROBLEM-PRODUCTION is that we need not concern ourselves with what is or is not reasonable. In fact, reason is one of the greatest enemies of PROBLEM-PRODUCTION.

It is not caution that we throw to the wind, but reason! When you firmly grasp that principle, very few things will be left standing between you and problems of whatever magnitude you wish to produce. Here are a few suggestions to get you started.

Create a phobia: Even a moderately creative person can generate an unreasonable fear of practically anything. Psychologists call some of these fears *phobias*. When one produces a fear in his or her life, he or she has a phobia. If one is afraid of closed places ("Kleiophobos" from the Greek) that person is the proud owner of *claustrophobia.*

A lot of fears have already been named for us; such as *acrophobia* (fear of high places), *agoraphobia* (fear of open places), *zoophobia* (fear of animals), *phobiaphobia* (fear of fear), etc. You need not, however, be limited to those already named and catalogued. It could be fun to make up and produce your own.

When your fear produces any one symptom, or any combination of several, you are having an anxiety attack. These attacks vary a great deal in different people, and even in the same person on different occasions. You may faint, have palpitations of the heart, be unable to breathe (temporarily), have assorted pains, or even, with some practice, break out in hives.

If you have the genius of a champion anxiety-neurotic, you can develop an unreasonable fear about anything. Exercise your genius. If you have it, flaunt it. Learn to fear bosses (bossophobia is a possible name, mixing English and Greek). You can learn to fear success, failure, going outside, staying inside, etc. Remember your fear does not need to be unusual, just unreasonable.

Two very clear benefits will become yours when you develop some really ridiculous fears. First, you can get a lot of attention and second, you can use your fear to avoid doing things you don't want to do. For example, you can startle people at large social gatherings by screaming, "I've got to get out of here, I've got claustrophobia."

Before going into more detail about developing fear, I should first caution you. Once you develop a fear and you want to keep it, *never test it*. Never face your fear. Testing is the quickest way to destroy most fears. One of my clients was suffering from acrophobia. On a trip, just before entering therapy, he had checked into a room on the second floor of a hotel. As he looked out the window he became so frightened that he crawled away from the window, cringing in speechless, helpless horror.

He extended his fear to include traveling across bridges. He said he "imagined himself flying off into space and became panic stricken." This never occurred close to home—it only happened on trips. He was a very insecure person and became frightened when facing change. He and his wife were planning to move—get this—to the mountains! This man did, however, honestly want to get rid of his problem.

He did two basic things. 1) He stopped saying ridiculous things to himself about flying off into space. He started saying to himself that these ideas were unreasonable. Rational thinking helped him to deal intellectually with his unreasonable fear. 2) On the practical level, he faced his fears. I went with him to high windows, and we looked out together. He overcame his fear and is presently living in the mountains with his wife.

Again, I emphasize, that if you are trying to develop a fear *you must not face it realistically.* Keep the consequences in your imagination. That's where they can do you the most harm. Reality testing is for the well-adjusted. *Don't test your fear if you want to keep it*, unless, of course, you're afraid of something like jumping from airplanes without a parachute.

For those of you who want to develop a fear and nurture it into a full-fledged anxiety, learning the following techniques is mandatory. Generalize from these examples to develop your own pet fears.

Use your imagination: Suppose you want to develop a fear of heights, acrophobia. You can start by imagining that you are falling. Close your eyes as you visualize yourself on a high mountain. Imagine that you feel the ground beneath your feet giving way, and visualize yourself falling through the air. Repeat this scene in your head over and over again until you feel it in your stomach.

In order to enrich your imagination, you will find that a library of reading material is helpful. Read all the news items you can find on air disasters and mountain accidents. Clip them, put them in a scrapbook or stick them on the bathroom mirror. With the combination of your own imagination and proper reading, you can scare yourself speechless within a few days.

The fear of heights will enable you to avoid all airplanes and mountain vacations and from going above the second floor in any building. If you really work at it, you can turn that fear into a reserve generalized fear—a sort of free-floating anxiety. You will be an anxiety attack looking for a place to happen. Then, when anything unpleasant faces you, you can produce a fear in order to avoid the occasion.

The beauty of unreasonable fear for skilled problem-producers is that it provides an excuse for failure in areas that aren't even related to that specific fear. You can fail at work, in marriage, in school, or even in sports, and blame it on your fear or anxiety. It is not at all improper to say, "If it were not for my acrophobia, I would have gotten those reports out on time."

Use it or you will lose it: Once you develop it, use it. The more often you use your fear as an excuse, the more securely entrenched it will become. Soon it will take an army of therapists to even uncover the roots of it. And without your cooperation, no one will ever be able to take it away from you!

Worrying about anxiety: Worry is as counterproductive and disabling as any other form of anxiety. *Worry is concern pushed to its illogical conclusions.* The best-adjusted people refuse to worry about things over which they have no control as well as about the things over which they do have control. So the best-adjusted people pretty much refuse to worry.

Nonworrying people say, "If I can't do anything about a situation it is a waste of time to worry about it. And if I can do something about a situation, I do it." That reminds me of my Dad's statement concerning the worry over money developed by roughly 97.3 percent of the population. He states simply, "If you have money, you don't need to worry and if you don't have it, you would spend your time better by going out to try to get some."

My father suggests that "worry" is a word that should be removed from the dictionary. He says, "That would stop the sale of a lot of tranquilizers. Most people only worry because they think they are supposed to, and if you removed that word, they wouldn't believe that any longer."

Of course, you can worry if you wish to worry. You can worry about anything. If you are producing anxiety, you can worry about that. Worrying will intensify your anxiety, and anxiety will increase your worry, and your increased worry will intensify your increased anxiety and ...

Turn criticism into catastrophe: Personally I find it easy to worry about or produce anxiety concerning criticism. Just the simple fact that we are alive means that we have been criticized by someone, somewhere, for something. Deduce from this that at this very moment someone either has or is about to be critical of you. It is obvious that you have enough reality to build an illogical network of worry. I have simplified the process with the following rules for turning criticism into catastrophe.

1. Assume that critics always know what they are saying. When someone makes a critical remark concerning you, say to yourself, "That person obviously knows what he/she is talking about so I had better take what he/she said seriously."

2. Fear the iceberg! This means that you say to yourself, "Usually people are so kind that they do not tell us how bad things really are, so if anyone says something critical to me, they must have left unsaid nine times more and worse floating beneath the surface." Such clever utilization of Titanic Fear enables you to turn every negative remark into a bitter condemnation.

3. Muse to yourself, "Now I have heard one person's criticism of me and, based on what I know about the sneakiness of people, that means practically everyone I know, plus a few strangers here and there, is criticizing me." Enters then the Titanic! You are on your way to sinking your ship with fear of all criticisms lurking below the surface. Never permit yourself to focus on reality. Control your urge to say, "Oh well, that is only one person's opinion, and it doesn't make a total wreck of my life to be criticized."

4. Borrow criticism from others. Don't waste valuable time just listening to critical comments concerning others. Apply the reverse Beasley Principle. Internalize those criticisms with a transitional thought such as, "That is more true of me than it is of Charlie." When you become skilled in transition, you will say to yourself, "That comment was probably meant for me anyway." When it comes to criticism, you can find an ample amount to supply yourself. But in the unlikely event that you run short—borrow from a friend.

5. Criticize yourself and assume that others agree. If you say it first, you will let others know what a realistic evaluation you have of yourself. You will ingratiate yourself by letting others know how clearly you see your own flaws, mistakes, errors, foibles, and warts. Obviously *they* noticed them first but were too polite to comment. Warning: There is a *slight* chance when you are just learning this technique that, from time to time, you will confront someone who disagrees with your negative self-evaluation and who will reassure you that you're not *that* bad. Pay no attention. It's easy to disregard. Someone is probably saying something critical about you even now as you read these words. The fact that you can't hear it does not mean it isn't there.

6. Never confront anyone who criticizes you in an effort to understand why or to clear up your own feelings. Go on being unrealistically imaginative about the criticisms heaped on you. Apply the techniques of Mountain Building and Negative Focus to all criticisms you receive.

Conclusion: Anxieties and irrational upsets are guaranteed if you will just practice the sincere, though at times somewhat absurd, suggestions I have given you in this chapter. Loft your sails in the winds of fear, worry and anxiety. Now lash yourself to the mast and look forward to a rough sea ahead.

9

Turning Decisions
Into Destructiveness
(Or How to Cop Out on Decision-making)

Decision making can be such a fertile source for PROBLEM-PRODUCTION, that it is too bad for people not to learn to use it thoroughly. Few people would deny that making decisions can be dangerous, even though those who behave responsibly make decisions as if decisions are a normal and necessary part of life. Therefore, if you are tired of the responsibility that comes from making decisions and prefer being viewed as indecisive and afraid, then you have an easily achievable goal. You need only three suggestions.

1. Think of danger: Remember and impress into your mind the fact that *decision-making can be dangerous*. There is always the possibility that you will make a bad choice. And no way of being absolutely certain that your choice will be a good one. Of course, life never comes with written guarantees. Though many people usually continue to live quite well, even after selecting bad options, don't let that fact deter you. Remember, when you are generating problems, you don't have to be reasonable. The fact is, it always helps if you can throw reason aside.

2. Extend the danger of major decision-making to include ALL decisions: The following story ended in an abortive action but the technique is valid. It would have worked if the woman involved had really wanted it to work. Even in PROBLEM-PRODUCTION some people resist. Seldom, however, does anyone resist as violently as one who is about to have problems taken away from him/her.

The client came to me because she was having trouble making the "big" decisions. It immediately became apparent that she did not really want to have help in accepting the responsibility for her decisions. She wanted to use her inability to decide as a means of enabling her to avoid decision-making altogether. She wanted other people to make choices for her. I actually recognized her resistance as I was pointing out the fact that most people make decisions and accept the hazards as "just part of living." She "just couldn't do that." I knew I had an opportunity to help her develop a neurotic fear of decision making—especially since she seemed to have a natural yen for excusing herself.

I began, "Why don't we wait a while to work on your problem?"

She continued, "Well ... I don't know ... why?"

It was obvious that the idea was not totally unwelcome, but she would have trouble deciding.

I continued. "Most of the people I see do not seem to realize how important and dangerous decisions can be. You are refreshingly different! You seem to have already learned how potentially devastating a bad option can be. I just don't believe you have pushed your thinking to its logical conclusion." (I could have said "illogical," but that would have defeated the whole process.)

She countered ambiguously, "How can I do that? ... I ... don't understand what you mean."

I pressed on, "Well, you have limited your indecisiveness to what you call 'big' decisions. Right?"

She hesitatingly replied, "Yes, I guess you could say that."

I asked, "Do you realize that all decisions may become 'big

ones?"

She made no verbal response, but by the way she was leaning eagerly forward, I knew she was interested. She may even have comprehended my reasoning process. Avoid making the "big" decision and you will become incapable of making any decisions. Once that is accomplished, there will be an end to the necessity of making choices of any size or consequence. You will become a robot whose control device is always in the hands of others.

I asked, "Are you willing to try something for one week?"

She indecisively responded, "I ... I guess so."

"OK. I want you to make a list of all the decisions you make during the normal course of one day. Start realizing that they are *all* major decisions. I'll tell you how it can work if you'll start keeping a record of what you say to yourself in order to reach that conclusion each time. I will use that information to help other people who want to develop an excuse in this area. I could even use it to help some people who want to develop the ability to *face* decisions."

She said, "I'll try." That was good enough, though I usually try to get a more firm commitment like, "Yes, I will."

I said, "All right, start when you leave this building. You probably know that there are two ways to exit the parking lot. Ordinarily you just drive off without thinking. Today I want you to sit in your car and tell yourself that this could be a vital decision. If you pick the wrong exit, you could have an accident that would have been avoided by going the other way. Or you might meet someone important to you if you do go in the right direction. Sit there until you decide you can take the chance or that you're willing to run the risk. (Some existentialists might suggest that she sit and think herself into the reality that there is actually no exit, much less a better one.) Go through that same thinking process at each intersection.

"Now when you arrive home, don't even turn on your lights without thinking. What if someone passes by, sees your lights on and stops to tell you something very important to your future? On the other hand, what if someone who will become a real problem to you stops in? You might be better off in the dark. Use this same process before you make any phone calls. The possibilities are endless."

She agreed to try it. We went over the instructions once more before she left to make sure she had them right. Her home was only about ten minutes from my office. More than an hour later my telephone rang.

She said, "I just got home. And I've changed my mind. This is stupid. I think I'd rather just go ahead and make decisions and let whatever happens happen."

I tried to hide my disappointment, "Well, that's your decision!" I had obviously pushed her too far. Still I have great faith in this technique and firmly believe that anyone who really tries can literally paralyze him/herself with anxiety about decision-making.

If you want to become neurotic and avoid responsibility for your decisions, work at the process I have suggested. If you apply this technique faithfully and find it ineffective, please contact me. On the other hand, if I hear nothing from anyone, I will know indecisiveness and procrastination have won the day. The point is, I don't want to know about success—only failure!

3. Start blaming others: Ask for and take advice from anyone. Then you have many handy scapegoats to blame when or if the decision is wrong. Hand over the responsibility for your decisions to others. Try to please everyone. Do just what others want you to do. Tell yourself that making decisions requires too much risk. Cop out!

10

This Will Make You Sick
(Using Emotions and Illnesses for Personal Benefit)

Just recently I discovered something I have known for most of my life. This probably means I have always been smarter than I am. My discovery, which no doubt has been known in one form or another by most people, is the fact that *we use our emotions and illnesses in ways that benefit us.*

When I was a small boy I learned that various kinds of sickness were very useful. A headache could 1) gain me a lot of attention and 2) help me get out of working or going to school. What I knew then, but didn't realize, was that I was developing very early an ability to use my emotions, as well as my physical illness, in ways that were advantageous to me.

By the time I was a freshman in high school I had convinced myself, my parents, and our family physician that I had a weak heart. I did this by hyperventilating, faking dizziness and falling back on the floor or ground as if in a dead faint. The doctor became so convinced that he advised my parents never to permit me to engage in any strenuous physical activities — including athletics!

In my fantasy world, I came to the realization that it would be very brave of me to risk my life by joining our track team and running the mile. My scenario included keeping my participation a secret from my parents and courageously gasping for breath as I crossed the finish line first, just before my weak heart gave out. I took the risk and ran for the wrong reasons. I may have been disappointed at first when I didn't drop dead and make them all sorry. But now as I look back, I'm glad nothing was really wrong with my heart.

I gave up on heart trouble because the cost of pursuing the malady (giving up basketball and track) was far greater than the rewards or the payment (getting out of working around the house). On a few occasions I have been tempted to return to the chest pain—for instance, when I'm watching television and my wife wants the trash taken out.

One Saturday afternoon when I was nine years old, I asked my mother and father if they would permit me to go to a movie. They both said, "No." I was heartbroken and immediately began to cry. I wanted to feel sorry for myself, and that was easier when I was alone so I hid behind our house. There I huddled by the wall and said to myself that it was terrible to miss seeing that movie. The more I wallowed in self-pity, the more I cried. In the midst of my tears, I began to fantasize. I imagined my father coming around the corner of the house, seeing me cry and feeling so sorry for me that he repented and offered to take me to the movie.

My fantasy didn't happen. But the idea was implanted. I could make good use of my bad feelings. I believe that a good many people say destructive things to themselves about their maladies. For example, "If they could see me now, they'd know how important it was to me." Or, "... they'd be sorry." Suicides sometimes even leave notes revealing their elaborate fantasies that after they die, the world will finally realize how much a relationship, a job, a sale or a victory would have meant to the poor victim.

In short, we tend to use our sicknesses for personal advantage. If we can discover why or how we use our problems, we can intensify the effect, if that is our desire. Or we can lessen the effect. Once a use is discovered, we can achieve the same effect through less painful means; for example, through *doing* the thing, seeking the job or person we were avoiding. It has been my experience that when such a course of action is followed, the disease or problem, no longer needed, often disappears.

It seems obvious that at the same time most of us are learning, early in life, that we can use our problems, *we also learn to generate them.* I believe that at least 85 to 90 percent of our problems are self-generated and can thus be dealt with effectively. What we produce, we can destroy or make over. If you want to become ill, follow these suggestions.

Imagination is always helpful: I am confident that you can make yourself sick. Read articles on specific diseases. Study the symptoms thoroughly. Once you are familiar with a disease, it is easy to imagine yourself sick with that particular disorder. If you practice imagining it long enough, you will be able to produce some real symptoms.

Scare yourself: In addition to imagining, you might try producing fear of a particular disease. This will force you to think about the disease, and you can easily magnify symptoms at that point.

At a biofeedback conference, I heard the following amazing true story:

A middle-aged man entered a hospital as an outpatient to have a benign growth removed from his face. The surgery was not serious enough to warrant a hospital stay. His physician finished stitching up the incision and left the office to discuss another patient with an M.D. colleague in the hall.

The hero of our story overheard the conversation and assumed that he was the subject of their conversation.

"The reports on your patient came back today," said the second M.D.

"Yes," said our hero's doctor. "I saw them—malignant."

"Yeah, it's a shame, too. It's my opinion that there is nothing we can do for him. I would not expect him to live out the year.

What do you think?"

"There is no doubt," said the hero's doctor, "that you are right. I don't know what to say to the family."

"Yes. That's sticky, a sticky one. Well, see you later."

The doctor stepped back into his office, somewhat pre-occupied (a condition interpreted by our hero as reluctance to talk about *his* condition).

Our patient was released. He never spoke of his "condition," but within a matter of a few weeks, he lost a considerable amount of weight. He developed severe pains, pains that would be associated with metastasized cancer. He soon had to be admitted to the hospital. He grew weaker and his condition became serious.

When his doctor expressed bewilderment, Mr. X bravely and weakly smiled, "You don't have to keep it from me. I know I have cancer. I overheard you talking to that other specialist after you removed the growth from my face."

After checking his calendar, the doctor was able to figure out what had happened. The whole situation was explained to Mr. X. It took some doing, but he was finally convinced.

The happy ending to the story is that the patient regained his health. The point for problem-producers to note seems as clear as the growth on your face. It's possible to dang nearly imagine yourself to death. And if you fully believe what you create, you can at least produce the symptoms of cancer itself. I believe we may soon discover that we can think ourselves into real cancer.

Perhaps another personal experience will help you to under-stand how this technique works, though I will confess that in my case this one was quite accidental.

A few years ago, I needed a physical examination to obtain a pilot's license. I went to the county health office for a chest X-ray and was informed that the results would be mailed to my home.

The following week my wife and children left town for a visit with some of her relatives, and it was my good fortune to receive the health service report on my physical condition while they were gone.

The letter came on Tuesday. I cannot remember the exact wording, but it went something like, "Dear Sir: Your X-rays indicate a need for further examination. You are scheduled for additional X-rays Wednesday morning at 9 a.m. There is no reason for alarm, but if you cannot make the 9 a.m. appointment, we advise that you see your personal physician at your earliest convenience."

I put the letter aside and pushed its contents from my thoughts until I went to bed. I laid down on the bed and turned off the lamp. Immediately, I felt a slight pain in my chest. My childhood symptom returned. It seemed to be getting worse. I was alone! I wondered if I should write a note with explanations and instructions in the event of my death. The telephone! I could call a friend and have him check on me the next morning. Panic! I could feel my "bum ticker" pounding. And then it occurred to me; the report could be wrong. And besides, there was nothing I could do about it.

I talked to myself a few minutes and prayed a child's prayer of commitment: "Now I lay me down to sleep. I pray the Lord my soul to keep. If I should die before I wake, I pray the Lord my soul to take."

Now I felt better and could laugh at myself. From then on I had no worry. And a week later I learned that there had been a speck of dirt on my original X-ray. I had no problem—but I nearly generated one. It would have been easy.

In reflecting on that experience, I realized that we all could contribute to our physical illnesses by using our fears and imagination. (I would imagine the process could be reversed, but that would begin to generate health, and we are still focusing on PROBLEM-PRODUCTION.)

You can make yourself sick, too. Think sick and become sick! Study disease! Learn symptoms. Watch every commercial on headaches, backaches, and hemorrhoids. Watch all medical shows on television. And don't forget to utilize magazine articles. Focus on your fear and use your imagination. All of this will make you sick.

Use your symptoms: When you want to hold on to a headache, permit that headache to become useful. Talk about how terrible you feel. Talk about all the things you would do or do better if only you didn't have that excruciating pain in your head. Mention the worst possible causes, like, "I sure hope this isn't a brain tumor." (Note that I am referring to everyday pains. There are certainly severe problems which anyone can recognize and check out through a physician.)

Create a symptom: One very clever symptom that one man created for himself was the existence of an almost constant fever. He convinced himself that his normal body temperature was 96.6. Every time his temperature checked out at 98.6, he had a fever of two degrees. Needless to say he had an almost constant fever. When his body temperature goes up to 101.6 degrees, he is near death, or as he says, "burning up with fever and nearly delirious."

If you need additional help, you might make a list of all the statistics you can locate which have to do with potential illness or problems. I have made some rough calculations. By adding together all of the things that affect 1 in 10, 1 in 20, or 1 in 5 people, I calculate that within the next year approximately 22 of every 10 people in America will be affected by heart disease, cancer, multiple sclerosis or mental illness, or will be the victims of violent crimes, auto accidents, plane crashes, fires or VD. Think about it. You can produce one of America's most prominent illnesses—fear. That makes me sick!

11

Developing Diversified Dependencies

(Comfortable Cop-outs)

No one blames a cripple for using a crutch. And in this canine-eat-canine world, we all limp a little at times. The fact is that life at its very best still requires enough effort and courage to create a little dread in us. So just say, "Of course I know I can make it, but even I need a little help. After all, I ain't perfect, am I?" Absolutely no one will accuse you of that, so you can begin immediate justification for something to lean on.

From justifiable concern and a desire for assistance, you can move into a state of useless, petrified fear and learn not only to lean on but live on your supports. Become addicted to something.

Following are a few simple steps toward making yourself into some kind of addict. I will also give you a list of things on which you can learn to rely and some specific examples to help you.

1. Think about the physical and emotional labor that will be required of you if you simply face life on your own. You may have to work at a productive job for many years to come. That thought alone should enable the average person to have at least a momentary yen for a "cop-out." Leave working to the

fools—you can find a better way.

You can have a lot of fun drinking or smoking pot or popping pills or watching TV. There are many choices that will enable you to escape reality—at least for a little while. Within no time, you can become an emotional cripple and discover a comfortable hiding place.

2. Refuse to listen to the advice of others—especially advice from people who seem to be fairly well-adjusted. Never, never listen to the advice of anyone who has worked through his or her problems. You have the right to produce and keep your own problems. Make your own mistakes.

3. Pay no attention to the warnings of researchers or professionals. Right away they'll have you assuming too much responsibility. At the very least look for a professional who will encourage you to dump the responsibility for your life on someone or something else (e.g., parents, society or environment).

Find someone to support your maladjustments and relieve you of any personal responsibility, with statements such as: "Your parents caused your condition by overprotectiveness"; "If your parents had not compared you to your siblings, you would not feel so discouraged."

4. Emphasize your weaknesses. Make the most of your inabilities. You'll feel better about becoming dependent on something if you can convince yourself you could never have made it anyway. "It is just as well that she got the promotion, I could never have handled that much responsibility anyway."

5. Use the stupidity of other people to justify your own stupidity. Never model your life after those who seem to be well-adjusted and effectively coping with life. Chances are, they are working, growing, and accepting responsibility for their own lives.

Perhaps you'll see what I mean more clearly in the following example:

I know a young man who has proved he is a genius at developing dependency. He began anesthetizing himself regularly on pot when he was fifteen years old. (You can start earlier if you want to really set yourself up for dropping out of life.) Now he stays stoned anywhere between 60 and 82.3 percent of his time. His biggest accomplishment thus far has been to show up for dinner.

Ten years ago I first talked to this young man and told him he was headed for emotional bankruptcy (I was naive at the time and thought he wanted something more than that). He was clever, though. He told me how ridiculous it was that I would suggest another style of life to him and informed me, "In the first place, marijuana is harmless. And even if it weren't, there are worse things." Now that is a neat thought! Etch it permanently into your mind if you want a dependency problem! "There are worse things!" Absolutely refuse—ever —to compare your behavior with "better things."

To justify your stupidity, you must compare yourself with people who are more stupid. This fellow is an expert. He thinks getting high on pot is better than getting high on alcohol. Now who can argue with that? It isn't absolutely necessary to cop out on anything but if you do, then never compare yourself with someone who is not copping out. To make such comparisons could ruin the whole process of PROBLEM-PRODUCTION. Only compare yourself with a person who is doing something at least equally as bad as what you are doing. You can follow this example in any behavior you choose. If you are getting drunk, it's better than being hooked on heroin. (Note the use of the words "better than." We all like to feel "better than" someone.)

6. Don't be choosey. You must maintain low standards. Use anything that is available to help you avoid facing reality, the enemy of anyone who wants to become dependent. You can become totally (almost) reliant on anything that enables you to avoid facing reality or avoid accepting responsibility.

Look at the following list of things you can lose yourself in. (Feel free to add to it. At least you can be creative about your dependency.)

Alcohol	Aspirin
Television	Another person

Sex	Cocaine
Heroin	Comics
Marijuana	Movies
Tranquilizers	Cigarettes (cigars or pipes)
Anti-depressants	"Red Devils"
Candy	Coffee
Food	Sodas
Therapy	Work

Of course some of these are much more powerful as dependencies than others. Some dependencies are supported only by psychological needs, while others enable you to develop genuine physical dependency. The vital action is to get so absorbed in whatever you choose that you have no time or energy left to devote to facing the realities of life.

TV-watching: Television is a convenient tool for dependency-seekers, because it is as harmless as a cocktail or a joint of marijuana. No one will ever accuse you of being immoral just because you watch television. Problem-producers know how to get the most from the most harmless things, and television is a good tool to use for an illustration. Its uses are almost unlimited.

1. You can use it to escape meaningful conversations. "Huh?" "Hey, can't you see I'm watching something?" "At least wait for a commercial break to begin talking."

2. Use it to escape thinking about the things you could be doing. You can almost lose touch with reality by becoming wrapped up in a story or program or until you are too sleepy to hold your head up; until your eyes burn so much you can no longer watch. Some escapees learn to lose themselves in the tube for up to 50 (or more) hours a week.

3. Use television to experience life vicariously. Live in a fantasy world and thus achieve all of your dreams without getting out of your recliner, except for drinks and "potty" breaks. Live in the fantasy land of the networks—avoid reality until the tube burns out!

4. Use it to intensify your own misery. Television soap

opera is the fastest active ingredient to bring on a sentimental heartache. Combine soap operas with the techniques you have learned in "The Art of Misery" and become miserable without even switching channels.

5. Use television as an excuse for avoiding anything you want to avoid. Watch the late shows and oversleep. Be late for work and blame television. Fail to do work and blame television. Learn to depend on television.

Drugs: Of course, most people look for something a little more exciting to use as a dependency. In America we love drugs. History will probably record that the second half of the 20th century produced millions of democratic-minded people who loved apple pie, the US of A, and drugs, both legal and illegal.

Depend on drugs for anything—acceptance, sleep, energy, temporary relief from everything and a ready-made excuse for malfunctionings of all types. However, there are several things you must do if you want to develop any kind of drug dependency:

1. Do *not* try to solve anything on your own. Remember, life is too much for you, and you've got to have help in order to survive. (This doesn't have to be true—you only have to convince yourself and make it true for you.)

2. Practice is a must. Occasional experimenting is not sufficient. It is all right for starters, but, as in any worthwhile project, one must practice in order to become proficient. Use your dependency over and over until you develop tolerance for the effects and a burning desire for support.

3. Assume that "everyone" uses them. How wonderful it is to be able to reinforce the rightness of what *you* are doing by having "everyone" on your side. In PROBLEM-PRODUC-TION peer pressure is one of the most powerful of all assistants, especially when it comes to developing drug dependencies.

4. Never yield to the temptation to stop once you start relying on drugs. If anyone should pressure you to quit, agree to do it but always at some future date. For example, one

counselee struggling with a dependency said she wanted to quit. I foolishly asked, "When?" She set a date all right, "July 30th." (It was January.) I could hardly resist asking, "What year?" but managed to restrain myself. Needless to say, she has managed to resist all efforts to overcome her dependency. Which leads me to this helpful suggestion if you are one of those who want to develop and retain drug dependencies: "Never quit today!"

Remember, any kind of dependency can offer you 1) a way to escape reality and 2) a way to avoid responsibility.

A lot of people develop dependencies on things they consider to be harmless. You can set yourself up for this move by convincing yourself that there is really nothing wrong with what you are about to do, in fact you will be *helped* by your new activity.

Once you convince yourself, you can effortlessly hold off others who try to "help" you overcome your habit. The following conversation involving a constant user of marijuana will illustrate the basic rationale and its application. "PP" is the problem-producer and "O" is his opponent. "O" could be a parent, friend, teacher or therapist.

O—"You sure have been smoking a lot lately."

PP—"Yeah, I enjoy getting high and I think life is too short to waste time being unhappy. I want to be happy as much as possible. (PP is convincing himself that happiness is not possible in reality, and, to him, temporary happiness is better than running the risk of facing reality.)

O—"Other people seem to be able to be happy without smoking anything."

PP—"Hey, that's their thing." (Meaning if I don't say anything about them, they have no right to say anything about me.) "Anyway, you shouldn't compare what I'm doing to anything that could include hard stuff—that's different." (Meaning "a crutch is not a crutch.") "What I'm doing is harmless and at least better than what others do." (Good move for a problem-generator. Recall that any comparison should always be stupidity with worse stupidity.)

O—"Well, I know what you're doing is not all that bad (you've got me) but you are beginning to spend too much time stoned out of your mind."

PP—"Come on, I know what I'm doing. I can handle it." (It always helps to assume omnipotence.) "Besides it's not a narcotic." (Another good move. This puts the problem into an area of debate. Note the argument moves away from the basic problem—dependency. Now O must either back off or begin a debate that goes nowhere.)

O—"Sure, but some experts are beginning to question the long-range effects ... (O has been pulled into the trap. He has been diverted by an expert.)

PP—"Bull! What do they know?—besides there are experts who disagree." (Essentially PP is saying, "Baby, you're in my ball park now and I never pay attention to people who disagree anyway.")

The discussion goes on, but it is pointless. When you want to develop a dependency, it helps to not deal with real issues. Discuss legalization of pot, the problems of others (alcoholics, heroine addicts, etc.), but always stay away from the issue of dependency.

The same basic approach is used for any dependency. Again, I don't mean to imply that they are all the same. Some are certainly more dangerous and destructive than others, but the way to get started on any of them is basically the same, since they all provide excuses for failure and ways to escape reality.

You can start with anything. Depend on pills for weight loss, tranquilizers for relaxation and sleep, anti-depressants for good feelings and energy, pills for easing headaches, etc. Most of these things could have good use and some people may use them wisely, but problem-producers use them in place of discipline and as a substitute for problem-solving or work.

Perhaps the three most important things to remember if you want to develop a dependency are:

1. Compare yourself with someone worse than you (they don't have to be *really* worse, just seem worse to you). I have discovered that most people have to feel "better than" before

they feel "as good as" other people. We have a tendency to want to feel *superior to* in order to feel *equal to* other people. This is illogical, but as we've shown, real logic has little to do with our lives.

2. Avoid looking at yourself honestly. Paint your own picture and disregard the opinion of others. Consensus may help discover scientific truth, but it gets in the way of PROBLEM-PRODUCTION.

One of my counselees kept telling me how awful she was, how unattractive, how unlikely to find a possible marriage partner. It never mattered to her that other people saw her in a more positive light. Once she told me, "Oh, I know that others disagree. Mary, John, Ted, Joy, my mom, my brothers, my sisters, a few others and you have told me I look nice and I'm a nice person. But·I don't believe any of you." I told her that was beautiful. Once your mind is made up, you need not be confused with the facts. (Of course, you can always change if you should decide at some future date that you can function better if you become more rational and responsible.)

3. Insist on doing your own thing; never pay attention to how your behavior influences your relationships with other people. Your selfish outlook will bring isolation, enabling you to pile on yourself a sense of rejection. Such rejection will prove that you need to lean on something. You probably recognize this as an application of the Pyrite Rule.

Workaholism: One of the most unique and ingenious of all dependencies is *addiction to work*. Workaholics are the people who always have more to do than they can possibly get done. At times such people seem to be striving for superiority. They never have time to deal with the issues of family life or social responsibility. They work, work, work, and the worst thing that happens to them is that occasionally someone will say, apologetically, "You are working too hard."

Imagine that! You can avoid facing responsibility, generate physical illness, excuse your failure (overloaded!), and people will feel guilty about being critical of you. Come to think of it—

you can work yourself to death, and people will say, "Poor guy (or gal), he (she) never took time for himself (herself). He (she) always took on the work load that should have been shared by others."

Most of us don't want to go as far as literally working ourselves to death—we just want a comfortable cop-out from the responsibilities of daily life. If you're looking for one of the most socially accepted cop-outs, with the possible exception of religious cop-outs, choose work. I suggest that it can be a very neat way of snowballing problems in your personal life, especially at home.

Workaholism can contribute to fantastically complex problems while simultaneously making you look like a saint. To develop this dependency, simply take on more than you can get done, stay late, take it home with you and add a part-time job.

This addiction dovetails nicely with marital problems. I know of people who have so successfully avoided responsibility that the only time they are seen at home by their families is when they eat (this can even be done on the job) or when they are sleeping. It will drive your spouse crazy if he/she is among the multitudes who are willing to cooperate by suffering in silence. This world contains enough spouses who are prone to suffer so that you probably can get away with practically any addiction you choose.

One type of person who can readily develop workaholism is the person who is easily duped into believing that he or she is essential to the world's continued existence. Try this on yourself. It can apply to any profession. Say, "My class cannot survive without me" or, "No one can make that sale but me." In essence, this line of thinking says, "I am absolutely vital to whatever job there is to be done." When you are honestly convinced of this you will be fully addicted and will probably need a tranquilizer for withdrawal.

The rationale for becoming a workaholic is simple. *Find value and worth not in yourself but in what you do.* This never proves anything, but it can certainly seem logical.

Learn to use one kind of work as an excuse for avoiding some other kind of work. This is a special adaptation of a psychological concept known as *substitution*. Also use work to escape facing reality. This trio of value, excuse and escape combine for a wonderfully harmonious foundation upon which to build workaholism.

Volunteeritis: One form of workaholism is so highly communicable that it should be classed as a social disease. I call it volunteeritis. It is a most ingenious form of escapism designed to snowball into maximum problems for the afflicted and a smorgasboard of problems for their families. It is a most clever malady in that all the while it is producing problems it is giving the appearance of social "do-goodism."

You can find allies in developing volunteeritis among highly respectable people, such as clergymen or charitable organization leadership. Other more suspect allies may be found among politicians on any level and, of course, among con artists who take advantage of anyone. For a limited time it is even possible to enlist the support of your family.

All you have to do is to stop accepting any portion of the responsibility for the daily functions arising in your family relationship, such as bill-paying, taking children to doctors or school functions, and house repairs. If you are unmarried or a student, stop social relationships, studying or whatever else requires your attention.

Now you are ready to start volunteering. Indeed a certain amount of volunteering *is* good. This fact, coupled with other problems, can give you ideal grounds for workaholism. Apathy is so widespread that most people won't care what you do—in fact, they will gladly let you usurp their share of any community responsibility.

But don't stop with civic responsibility and responsible concern. Push on to better things. You'll be praised for it, and, for a limited time, your family or friends will feel guilty if they criticize you.

Volunteers are in demand everywhere. Branch out. Start

with jobs that really need doing, and then leap into any group that gives you a badge, button, banner, chair to sit in, place to stand, letter to write, phone to dial or answer, literature to hand out, beads to count, toothpaste to test, cheese to taste, birds to inventory, leaves to collect or wild animals to round up for the ark. Strangers will admire and love you, while your problems snowball and your real responsibilities pile up like an avalanche of manure on your family and friends.

You may someday be crowned Volunteer of the Year. Such an honor will enable you to feel total rejection and misunderstanding from unappreciative children and friends, who during your absence have been compelled to assume your legitimate responsibilities. You are now a prime candidate for depression because you have no one with whom to share your hour of glory. They have all departed to other mates, stepparents or friends or may be convalescing in a rest home. Now you not only have problems; you *are* a genuine problem and are ready for VA (Volunteerics Anonymous).

Please note that volunteer work is not the cause of volunteeritis. Volunteers are needed and do a lot of worthwhile things. More genuinely concerned people are vital to useful organizations.* I point to these healthy helpful volunteers not only to admit the truth but to give all you problem-producers some additional grounds to excuse your blooming workaholism. These are some basics—if you want a problem, work at it!

---

*I emphasize this fact because I am still actively seeking people to work in church activities and educational projects. Just call me if you should have a few hours to fill.

·

12

Alcohol, Our Old Friend and Buddy

Of all the people who may read this book, alcoholics need it least. They are probably more skilled and knowledgeable in PROBLEM-PRODUCTION than I will ever be. Alcoholics, and the thousands of freeloaders who claim to be alcoholics as an *excuse* for their drinking, have developed techniques which can be invaluable to problem-producers.

Problem-producers can even learn to push a little truth further by listening to alcoholics, their families and the treatment people and researchers who earn their living from alcoholics and government grants for the intoxicating study of the growing malady of alcoholism.

I will now reveal to you secrets that will enable you to stay off the water wagon and jump on the bandwagon. You can be an alcoholic—or at least fake it enough—to make not only your life miserable but generate misery for everyone in your family.

Let's Make Alcoholism Unanimous

So you want to be an alcoholic? It must be easy to do, because we now have more than nine million of them in this country.

Americans have promoted this problem to the point that it now ranks as the Number Three Killer in this country. You can do it if you can take the ultimate pain. (I will admit to you that this is a journey that has a painful destination, but it may be worth it. After all, you get what you pay for, and the more intense problems cost more!)

Push the truth: (This is very similar to stretching the truth.) People who become alcoholics and those who cooperate with them are experts — *The Experts* — in this technique. I will give you only a partial list with comments that clarify their approach.

1. Alcoholism is a disease. This is true. It is inhumane to reject the disease concept of alcoholism because such rejection makes it more difficult for real alcoholics to face themselves. True! Now for the push: People who are diseased cannot help themselves. This helpless stance will allow you to excuse yourself from seeking treatment. Ignore your responsibility and choice to stay away from alcohol even if you are somehow manipulated into treatment and become sober. If you have a slip or relapse (and relapse is characteristic of the disease), give up, prove you can't help yourself (even though hundreds have made it to sobriety after slipping).

If you are dry, you can get hooked again by one good stiff drink and then moan, "Must be my old disease acting up again."

2. Real alcoholics are addicts. True! They are physically dependent on alcohol. True! This means you can never drink again if you want to recover. True! Now for the push: Say, "I can *never* drink again." Say it with pathos and hit "never" very hard. Act as if this constitutes a major tragedy. How can you live without drinking booze! You are the victim of a unique catastrophe. Never mind the diabetics who can never eat sugar or who have to take insulin regularly. Never mind asthmatics who can't run. Never mind other diseases that necessitate abstinence from various things. And for God's

sake ignore recovering heroin addicts. They will have to live without heroin. But things like heroin, sugar and air are not as essential to life as drinking. After all, you can wail pathetically, "Everyone drinks."

3. Real alcoholics will never be cured. True! Once an alcoholic, always an alcoholic. True! But push it: Convince yourself that this means you will never change in any way. Use this as a justification for any hang-up you want to keep. When you manage to justify complete stagnation in all personal growth, you can learn to depend on groups for your support. Avoid constructive groups, which grow along with the people in them. Instead, find yourself a group that has become ingrown and stagnant, where the same problems are rehashed for years and where the level of maturity remains the same. Such unchanging groups may produce another form of addiction—groupaholism. Thus, group support pushed to its extreme can become group cop-out.*

4. There are no known-for-certain characteristics that enable anyone to identify an alcoholic personality. Alcoholics can only be identified through their drinking habits. True! Push it and keep on pushing it: It is so difficult to determine a real alcoholic from one who claims to be one that treatment people have just broadened the circle to include more and more people. There are supposed to be at least four types of alcoholics and at least a dozen variations of each type. We may soon blur the lines so much that if you live near a bar, you will qualify for treatment programs.

Or even if you are not an alcoholic, you can drink enough to claim alcoholism. You will then be associating with the problem-producers who are the envy of all other problem-producers, those with no distinguishable characteristics, whose problems have no known cause!

---

*Please note that anyone who feels the need of a group should never deny him/herself that support through fear of groupaholism. It is a lesser addiction. Besides, who knows when, with the addition of a new member, a new experience, a new insight or concept, a group may start growing again. (It's a long worm that never turns!)

5. Alcoholics are usually good con artists. This is true! Just remember if you are worth six cents as a con artist, I have just given you four cunning conning tools. Truth is pushed too far when you can proudly say, "I am a *con*fessed con. I even con myself."

Push the lie: Turning lies into apparent truth is not as creative as stretching truth into lies, but it is effective. I will list some of the standard lies of alcoholics. You can use them for starters. Then if you need more help, attend an open meeting of an AA group, where you can learn from recovering alcoholics the lies they formerly pushed.

1. *Deny that alcohol is ever a problem to anyone, especially you:* When you begin to get drunk frequently, you notice your pattern of drinking changing, becoming less predictable. Ignore these warnings. No matter how many family members and friends notice the problem—deny! Conceal excessive drinking, sneak drinks if you must, learn to *act* sober—just *never* admit to yourself or anyone else that you have a drinking problem.

2. *Blame someone else for your drinking:* When your drinking pattern becomes obviously serious, refuse to accept personal responsibility. You can always find someone or something to blame. You drink because people put too much pressure on you at work. You drink because your family doesn't understand you or love you. You drink because the people in your neighborhood hassle you. You drink because of financial problems. You drink because your parents failed to teach you how to cope with life's problems. You drink because your religion has failed you. You drink because it is raining. You drink because it is not raining. You drink because the weather is hot or cold or in between. You drink because it is January, February, March, April, etc. The important thing is that you drink because ... *Never* admit that you drink because you choose to or because you do not choose to do anything about it.

It is helpful to have excuses. There are many things or people you can blame without ever having to admit that you are responsible for your own behavior. A hopeless spouse makes the most convenient excuse. "My wife nags at me," or, "My husband never pays any attention to me."

Employers run a close second and can be confused with your job responsibilities. "They expect too much out of me. It is not humanly possible to do all that they expect." "There is so much pressure on this job I just can't take it without a drink or two."

Some alcoholics blame their children. "They're always yelling." "This generation just expects too much." Remember you have a chance not only to excuse yourself but to generate almost insurmountable problems for your children at the same time.

Your excuses need have no connection with reality. You can blame your friends, the neighborhood in which you live, the world situation, your dog or even your car. The main point is that if you want to keep your problem, you must avoid accepting responsibility for it yourself. Just be sure to say "It's not *my* fault that I drink," after each new drinking experience.

3. *Tell yourself you must drink to relieve tension:* Just to be sure you always have an excuse to drink, drink to relieve tension. This is safe, because you can always produce tension. You can get tense at work, at home, at a ball game, watching television, driving, flying, swimming. You can produce tension in yourself by thinking of the dangers to your health from smoking, danger to your life from breathing, danger in crossing streets, danger of nuclear war, danger of falling meteors, danger of your spouse leaving you, danger of your children becoming dope addicts (I think that is the most interesting of all for alcoholics to be tense about—one addict worrying about someone else becoming an addict), danger of the sky falling. Tension is easy to create. Drink to relieve it. It will never work, but it is a dandy excuse for drinking.

4. *Tell yourself social drinkers drink alone:* Claim to be a social drinker, and then drink alone. If anyone asks you about this, tell them it is still social drinking because you think about people while you drink. That makes it social, doesn't it?

Keep on denying: Alcoholism starts with denying and continues with denying. Denial is essential to alcoholism. Deny with love. Deny with anger. Deny and appear to be hurt that anyone could think you have a drinking problem. Deny while crying. Scream your denials and shake your fist. Deny. Deny. Deny. Once you admit a need for help you are on your way to losing your problem.

Hang on to your old buddy. For tension, for comfort, for company, for easing your pain, for courage and for fun, grab that old bottle. It is a friend to the end—and it can even help you find the end!!

You can really dramatize the possibility of dying from alcoholism. Statisticians have given you a wonderful tool to use in producing guilt and fear in anyone who dares to question the validity or seriousness of your drinking problem. Say, "You realize, of course, that 36 of every 38 alcoholics die without having been diagnosed." They will be clouded by so much guilt and fear that they will never even think to ask, "Who finds and counts the undiagnosed alcoholics?" Personally, I suspect the figure is more like 87 of every 89, but regardless of the actual numbers, you can be one.

Plan to fail (The "I told me so syndrome" applies here): When you are cornered and have to admit that you are an alcoholic that is not the end. It is easy to *make promises* and easier to break them. Anyone can "fall off the wagon." You can fail as often as you choose.

You can Play the Game, Too
(For Families of Alcoholics)

If you are married to an alcoholic, you may have felt upstaged by him/her. Your problems seem dwarfed in comparison. You may even have been able to kid yourself into believing you are healthy. The chances that a really healthy person will marry an alcoholic are probably less than one in 812.

Even though you have produced serious problems for yourself, you may need help in clarifying them. This chapter is intended not only as instructions for further PROBLEM-PRODUCTION, but also as a magnifying glass through which you can see the actual enormity of the problems you already have.

1. You probably married a sickie because your own self-concept was so poor that you either believed no healthy person would ever be willing to stoop low enough to marry you or you wanted someone you could relate to as an equal. You may even feel better than your spouse. Remember that many people, perhaps you, have to feel *better than* before they feel *equal to* others.

You have a fantastic opportunity to reduce your already staggering self-concept. Tell yourself that if your spouse really loved you he/she would stop drinking for you. The fact that they have not means they do not love you. Now say, "If a drunk doesn't love me, no one else will." Feel the despair of being that unworthy! Dig yourself a pit in the valley of self-deprecation and crawl into it. You have done the best you could, and look at what you have.

2. You probably married someone who really needed a strong person (or at least a person) to help him/her get life pulled into shape. You have offered yourself as the rescuer, and now the rescuee has failed to respond to your efforts. Tell yourself that you are a failure. If you can't help someone you love, you can't help anyone at all. Apply the Reverse Beasley Principle. Blame yourself for your spouse's problem, and make it your own.

3. You are at least a latent martyr, if not a practicing one. In order to force this tendency into your life, you must continue to tolerate whatever abuse you have been called upon to suffer. Such suffering is most effective when done in

silence. Tell yourself that you are like an innocent, dumb sheep being lead to the slaughter. (Don't forget that *dumb* means more than just silent.)

4. Tell yourself that you innocently married an alcoholic. If you had known, you would never have been so foolish. I had one client who had divorced her third husband because he was a hopeless alcoholic. "Coincidently," her first two husbands were as alcoholic as her father. Why did she come to see me? She wanted me to talk to her present fiance. Would you believe he is an alcoholic?

She is an expert at PROBLEM-PRODUCTION, so she will continue to tell herself that it is all "happen-chance." So can you.

I do not mean to imply that mates of alcoholics are consciously aware of all or any of these things. Some people honestly want to face and overcome their own unhealthy tendencies. Such people will probably find a treatment group. Problem-producers do not follow those people.

What if Someone Gets Your Goat

There is no need to panic, but it is possible that you could suffer a temporary loss of your problems. Alcoholics do recover and spouses do grow. The old problems may be lost. It is like outgrowing a favorite dress or suit. Remember what you did in those circumstances? You bought a larger size.

Every family needs someone or something to blame for their problems. So you do need some suggestions for emergency action in the event that you lose your scapegoat.* If your alcoholic goat recovers, you need only have a minor dilemma.

1. During the transition between the outgrowing of old problems and the production of larger-sized ones, you can use preownaynictgut thinking. Blame one another for the bad old

---

*Animal used by ancient Israel to carry their sins out of their camp. We use the word to indicate someone or something to blame.

days. Unleash your pent-up anger, resentment and hostility. This will keep things tense while you regroup.

2. Look for a new goat. Creative families will audition scapegoats, i.e., try out several new ones and decide on the best of all candidates. I strongly recommend some sort of auditioning process, because the hit or miss technique frequently leaves us with a very poor substitution. A poor choice forces us into taking responsibility for some of our own problems and most of us certainly don't want that. No self-respecting problem-generator wants to take the responsibility for his or her own problems.

It may not be as difficult as it first seems. You may not have to do any auditioning at all. Frequently someone will volunteer for the part. Many families have would-be martyrs lurking in their closets. When difficulty arises, they are the ones heard muttering, "It's all my fault. I just mess everything up." In the family of an alcoholic, these people frequently have played a supporting role. It is almost impossible to upstage an alcoholic, so they just admit that they are one of the reasons for the drinker's problems. When the alcoholic begins to deal with life in a healthy way, they have their chance for the spotlight.

If no one volunteers and you have no desire to assume the role yourself, you can run tests to find the most talented prospect. One by one you can encounter the other members of your family by saying something like, "Now everything would be fine in this family if you would just get your head on straight."

The best candidate for blame will immediately internalize what you've said. This person will frequently blush and look away or if he or she is a ready candidate for manipulation, burst into tears. You must select the one who has the most apparent weakness.

If you are really at a loss and are fortunate enough to have teenagers, they make near-perfect scapegoats. I've known of some teenagers who are so gullible that they will accept the responsibility for major conflict between their parents and various family problems. They are almost defenseless because:

a. Most of them are easy to manipulate into rebelling. All you have to do is put a little pressure on them to cooperate with the rest of the family, and they, being eager to "establish a separate identity," will usually fall into the trap. See the chapter on the generation gap.

b. Everyone knows that teenagers are rotten trouble-makers anyway. You can accuse them openly and very few people would doubt it. Their own insecurity will make them so defensive they will soon look guilty or even become guilty.

c. They enjoy attention and most of them get so little that they'll be willing to suffer a bit just for the attention, even if it is negative.

Remember that, by the time most alcoholics have become honest enough to face themselves as alcoholics, the whole family has become infected by the disease. There usually is enough built-up hostility and resentment to last for years. As a result of the denial by the alcoholic and the cooperation of other family members, almost anyone in the family can produce a problem of his/her own or accept responsibility for the problems of others (which is a sneaky way to develop a problem).

Members of recovering alcoholic families may assume guilt for present feelings of anger or resentment toward one who is recovering no matter what the source of that anger or resentment. Or they may still blame themselves for the former problems.

3. If there are no available scapegoats, you can squeeze back into the old problems. With enough discouragement most alcoholics are willing to stumble back into drinking again. There are advantages to this move. It enables you to produce a new sense of failure. "I guess I'm just no good and never will be."

You can find alcoholic literature to support you in failing by suggesting that most alcoholics must fail three or four times. By the time you, the alcoholic, and you, the spouse, work through two or three failures, you may be lucky enough that one of you will be dead or just gone. The remaining spouse will not need me to explain how to use such a circumstance to produce guilt and bitterness.

The loss of a goat is not fatal. Look for a new one, and remember the old goat may come back at any time.

13

In the Name of God!

Over the years "religious" people have done every imaginable —and occasionally a nearly unimaginable—thing in the name of God. Rarely has a war ravished a country or the world that people on one side or both were not out there killing one another in the name of God.

In the name of God, people have been crucified, whipped, stretched (sometimes by the neck), burned at stakes, stoned to death and often even treated inhumanely. It should come as no surprise to anyone that religion can be used to help people produce problems.

The principles in this chapter can be adapted by any religion. I just happen to be more familiar with the Christian religion. As a pastor I have had many opportunities to help people develop serious problems, but teachers of religion and laymen, as well as pastors, can all contribute.

I have some advice for fellow churchmen and others in a position to aid those of us who wish to continue the fine tradition of contributing to PROBLEM-PRODUCTION. It is this —we must recommit ourselves to the Negative Trinity of Guilt, Rejection, and Fear.

1. Guilt-inducement is the easiest to achieve. Because we all make mistakes, we are all vulnerable to any suggestion that we are bad people. Clergymen can talk about all the things people should do but can't—plus all the things they shouldn't do but must—and thus leave their parishioners feeling frustrated and guilt-ridden.

Saturate your sermons, lessons and admonishments with statements such as, "You are terrible. You should know better. You must be perfect, but you're not." We can make people so conscious of all the possible negative actions they do or might do that they will believe their only hope rests in lying down and becoming very still.

Avoid the temptation to focus on grace and love, and never mind encouragement. Such things help people to overcome problems, not produce them.

2. Making people feel rejected is almost as easy. Most people are so afraid of being unacceptable that the slightest innuendo insinuating that they are unfit for fellowship with "good" people will be picked up immediately. We must avoid the tendency to separate the sin from the sinner; otherwise the church will be overrun with social and moral renegades. Let us hold the standard so high that few indeed will dare to feel accepted. As long as we do this, no one will ever be able to accuse us, as they did Christ, of associating with publicans, sinners and winebibbers.

Let the sinner find his acceptance among the sinners. We can keep our skirts clean and at the same time help generate a terrible sense of rejection in the masses of human wrecks who need help. We can turn our churches into museums for saints and spiritual relics. We dare not run the risk of permitting unclean and sick people to come into our fellowships. They might be accepted and think they are welcome among us. A rejecting attitude will assure us of a continuing place in the PROBLEM-PRODUCTION Hall of Fame.

3. The final characteristic in this trinity is fear. If we can convince people that they should be afraid of our God, surely

they will not come boldly into His presence expecting love. I have heard some preachers and teachers who are so skilled at producing fear that they can make many of their hearers afraid to go to the bathroom, lest they be caught there when the final curtain comes crashing down. No one wants to be found in the john at the end of the age.

A friend of mine who was a bus driver for many years told me that bus drivers would be awarded a higher position in heaven than a lot of preachers because they scared more hell out of people in one ride than the latter did in dozens of sermons. He has caught the spirit of a good many religionists who traffic in fright.

If we can add to the trinity listed above a strong conviction that we know everything there is to know about truth, we will not have to run the risk of being questioned. And we'll drive away all those truth-mongers who raise embarrassing questions with which they threaten to turn the altars (which have become judgment bars) into havens of refuge for the seekers of solutions and honest answers.

Admittedly, our ranks have been infiltrated by some of these well-intentioned, but obviously ignorant, people who think we ought to be contributing to solutions rather than problems. Still I am not afraid for the relative safety of the fortress because there are so many church leaders who are stubbornly committed to PROBLEM-PRODUCTION for churchgoers.

If you are a churchgoer you may have lucked into one of those fellowships where acceptance and love are preached with only an essential warning of the natural consequences of running from God's love. If so, you may be having trouble developing problems. Do not despair. Look for another church...

Look for a congregation that always dots every "i" and capitalizes every Don't. (If you remove "don't" and "shouldn't" from the manuscripts or notes of a great many preachers, priests and rabbis, you'd have a lot fewer complaints about long sermons or lessons.) Once you've found the "right" congregation, produce guilt in yourself by selecting any one of their hundreds of "don'ts" and doing it. Follow this by saying to yourself "I'm terrible. I shouldn't have done *that*." You can add others' rejection of you to your problems by being honest and open about the "don'ts" you've done.

Let me illustrate how bad the situation is by telling you about a couple who came to talk to me recently about conflict in their marriage. After confessing to their imperfection, they looked silently at the floor and then quietly said, "I guess this means you won't want us to come to church." They would be surprised to know that some churches actually accept imperfect people—drunks, divorcees, adulterers, adulteresses, homosexuals, alcoholics, gossips, tightwads, bores, pharisees and even a few speeders and income tax frauds. Not only do they accept them, they encourage them to stay and become whole. If you run into one of these crazy congregations, get out and try the church down the block. Churches welcoming imperfect people are so rare you are not likely to run into two of them in the same neighborhood.

Those of us who are committed to PROBLEM-PRODUC-TION can take great comfort in the fact that we will seldom be opposed by religionists. They are busy guarding orthodoxy, upholding tradition and blending into the current scene. They will not find much time to deal constructively with human problems.

14

Simple Sins for Individual Saints

I am particularily fascinated with the way individuals use religion to generate problems. These following remarks are not intended to be a put-down to genuine religious faith nor to the many honest and sincere adherents to various faiths. Though the principles set forth here may be applied by any religious sect, as earlier indicated, I have learned them through participation and observation in the Christian faith.

One of the fundamental principles in PROBLEM-PRODUCTION is the *denial system*. Although alcoholics may well be the leading specialists in the use of denial, I'll wager that the people of most religious groups run a very close second.

In case you haven't already figured it out, let me help you by pointing out the fact that any of your own private viewpoints can be validated by religion. You can be a racial bigot or a racial purist, a teetotaler or a social drinker, a prostitute or a client of same, a pacifist or a war-monger, and find support for your views in some religious and sacred writings.

The Bible itself can be used to prove, for instance, that any act *I* commit is pure (virtuous). Titus 1:15 says, "Unto the pure all things are pure." It can also be used to prove that any act *I* don't like (usually what *you* do) is wrong. In Romans 14, the same author says anything that causes offense to another is wrong. In other words, any act can be viewed as wrong if it is offensive to anyone and any act can be viewed as pure if the actor is pure in motive.

To get into this kind of game-playing, you have to move away from great principles of religion and get into hair-splitting, but anyone can do it. Such extreme questions as "Who caused David to take a census in Israel, God or Satan?" can be pursued. Both answers are clearly given in the Bible (2 Samuel 24:1 and 1 Chronicles 21:1). Now do you get the picture? You can do or believe almost anything you want and find some proof for it, so you are free to use religion to help in problem-generation.

Let's get back to denial (a form of snowballing at times), which is a basic tenet for those of you who want to get serious about developing problems within your church as skillfully as you develop them in other areas of your life. Religion offers some excellent aids for denial:

1. First, you can deny the existence of all evil. This can be promoted as a logical consequence of the existence of a good God. The argument is that God created all things; God is good; therefore, he created no evil things. If evil cannot exist, then it cannot be true that you have any problems. You can hang onto this denial until you reach the bottom of the hill. At that point, your problems will mangle you, and all anyone will need to hear from your lips is one final assertion of your basic philosophy, as from under the wreck you cry out, "Good God!"

2. A second way of denying is to admit the existence of problems, but deny that you have any responsibility for dealing with them. You will now not only be able to build problems for yourself, but also contribute to the problems of others.

When someone seeks your counsel or help, feed them the old denial system, as in:

Seeker: "Brother can you help me? I've lost my job, my house burned down, and ..."

Holy problem-producer: "Well, praise the Lord, my friend, that's a wonderful chance to demonstrate the power of your faith." (This not only insists that the seeker deny all problems, but it makes him or her feel guilty if he or she doesn't.)

A few things in the New Testament will have to be rearranged if you want to use them to support your denial system. You can begin by *proof texting** the commands to always rejoice and trust—then rewriting certain key sections. In order to justify your view that there is never any justification for sorrowing or feeling sad you have to remove or explain away examples of sorrow and sadness.

When you discuss Christ in the Garden of Gethsemane, don't picture him as struggling with the reality of the cross or death and rejection. Picture him as smiling, waving his hands, and praising the Father as he tries to pep up his sleepy band of disciples. Ignore what is reported as His genuine struggle and pain.

You can change the scene where he sat crying over the city of Jerusalem to a scene where he is totally unaware of rejection. Picture him as sitting there—alone, with a sheepish smile, humming hallelujahs to God. (A lot of denyers wear sheepish smiles.) Make him appear to be immune to or unaware of being rejected.

Some people use a similar technique for inspirational purposes, with basically the same erroneous results. I call it the "fall-and-point" system. Let the Bible *fall* open, close your eyes and *point*. The hope is that you'll find the exact right thought for yourself.

The classic example concerns a very depressed person who let the Bible fall open, pointed and read, "He went out and hanged himself."

---

*Using proof texts is a religious counterpart to the use of statistics. As you know, one who is skilled in the use of statistics can prove practically anything by making a selected reference to some statistic. The practice of taking statements out of context and using them for evidence is an art that has been employed by religionists since early April of 4004 B.C.

A second fall-and-point was utilized, and the depressed read, "Go and do likewise."

Not satisfied with the "divine" guidance received in the first two attempts, once more the fall-and-point was used. This time a shaking finger fell on, "Whatsoever you do, do it quickly."

Proof texting, then, is used to prove anything one wishes to prove by citing chapter and verse out of context and claiming such evidence as a clear indication that you agree with God or (more likely) that God agrees with you.

3. Denial, like schizophrenia, has many faces. A third way it appears is in the form of *pious and humble confession of success.* "I do not mean to boast—God knows I have no right to boast—*but* I was able to respond with grace and love to my absolutely paganistic, insensitive and vulgar boss. The most fantastic part of my ability to be calm was that he/she was reading me the riot act because of something I had not even done." The skilled denyers will follow this statement by looking at the floor and frowning as if there is mud on his or her shoes. And then slowly sit down, keeping the head lowered.

For problem's sake, please note that you are to confess only successes—*never confess failures.* Share with friends, publicly when possible, as many of your success stories as you can. Tell of the drinks you resisted, the temptations you overcame, the kindnesses you personify, the pounds you lost. It is even a nice stroke of public relations if you give God partial credit. Do not balance these "confessions" with reality. Do not mention slipping in temptation, taking a drink (falling off the wagon), or gaining a few pounds (falling on the table).

This lopsided confessional also will contribute to the problems of honest people. If any honest people believe you, they will withdraw from your religion either because 1) yours is a form of religion far removed from the world of success *and* failure where they live, or 2) they will feel so inferior to such a "purely" successful religionist as you are that they will simply give up.

I have called this third form of religious denial the three-in-one denial or the *trinity of denial.* It has *three* advantages for problem-producers. By being open about goodness and closed about badness, you create a public image beyond your potentiality. You are thus assured of failing (*assured failure* is the first problem). By creating a false image you have become a practicing hypocrite. This can be used to generate guilt feelings (*guilt feelings,* the second problem). And by contributing to an atmosphere that turns honest people away from you, you have assured yourself of some rejection (*rejection,* the third problem and final member of the denial trinity of problems).

Perhaps the most clever and demonic of all irresponsible denials is the use of religion as a dependency. (The general development of dependency is discussed in the chapters on "Developing Diversified Dependencies" and "Alcohol, Our Old Friend and Buddy.") Multitudes of people have discovered that they can avoid facing reality just as effectively by hiding behind religion as they can by using drugs (some use both in combination, i.e., the generation of "religious" experience with hallucinatory drugs or the use of tranquilizers and anti-depressants to make it through the week between religious meetings).

I know of people who have perfected this system to the point that they can spend hours—days—even weeks and months in one kind of religious meeting or another. They sing, they pray, the hug, they shout. And when their neglected friends or families desert them, they feel persecuted and use pseudopersecution as a further vindication of their "faith." This enables anyone to feel holy about the whole rotten process of PROBLEM-PRODUCTION. Clever?

I have stupidly fought this tendency in myself and others at times. I periodically fall into the trap of believing that good people would better exhibit their faith by being out working with suffering humanity and attempting to correct social injustices. Of course, that always necessitates inconvenience, sacrifice and action. Surely the churches would be a lot more full if we spent less time making love to ourselves (a form of spiritual masturbation) than trying to get out there and make love to a difficult world.* And we do measure truth in terms of success and numbers, don't we?

Of course, religion frequently is used to solve problems, and for honest seekers, that is a valid use. A lot of people are very good at this process, but that's for another book and another time. Let's just keep our focus on how to develop those problems. Praise the Lord! Amen!

---

*Note: People who have already developed personal skills in the use of religion in problem-production should be feeling a sense of "righteous" indignation from reading this. You should be able to either feel a keen sense of persecution because you are so horribly misunderstood or you should be locked into a total denial system that will enable you to reject all that has been said as meaningless and impossible. If you have had neither of these reactions you may need to apply the Reverse Beasley Principle and reread this section. If you are unfortunate enough to have a balanced approach to religion that involves both devotion and action, you may have trouble developing a significant problem through the use of religion, so go on to something else.

15

Counterproductive Living

Some men and women, thousands annually, decide against life in a very hostile and dramatic way. They kill themselves. Obviously people willing to go that far are either so angry or feel so worthless they can no longer think. Many of them probably could think if they wanted to, but they choose to take a cheap shot at life and the people around them. Ridiculous! There are far more effective ways to cop out on life.

If you don't choose one of the many addictions to neutralize your life and excuse yourself from productive living, you can take a most subtle and fantastically effective way out of useful living. You'll even be able to stay around and enjoy the frustration this will bring to your family and others in your society.

The technique is one that will have particular appeal to intellectuals, spiritualists of various kinds and, especially, those who are philosophically oriented. It can, however, be used by anyone.

I have named this technique for avoiding present responsibilities "counterproductive living." It could probably be called "counterproductive thinking" just as accurately because it is scarcely living at all, and thus is a much better solution to facing life than suicide or addictions to dangerous drugs.

I will describe for you the four basic components and demonstrate simple applications. Then I will demonstrate how they can be used in combination with each other to produce what I technically call "double-bind counterproduction."

1. The first technique is called, in layman's terminology, "regretting the past." If this were a psychology textbook, this technique would be called *"preownaynichtgut."**

You can easily perfect this method of escaping present living, but it does require a specific use of negative focus. To use this method effectively you only have to remember how tough you have had it in the past. Remember the hard times. Remember the missed opportunities. Bemoan the fact that you were born in an underprivileged family, poor family, rich family, overprivileged family or that you really had no family. Complain to yourself and others that you were mistreated as a child, spoiled as a child or never really treated as a child.

Remember how your brother, sister, friend or enemy always got the breaks you actually deserved. Fate not only frowned on you—she screamed obscenities at you. Fantasize that you could have been wealthy, powerful, maybe even a king or a president if you had only_____ .
Be creative and fill in the blank in whatever way appeals to your favorite fantasy.

A good example might be, "I could have been an honor student, gotten a scholarship to college, etc., if I had only studied more." Or "hadn't had to work so much" or "if the seventh grade math teacher had liked me."

Don't slip up and get caught utilizing the past as a lesson to help you live better now. Just think about it; focus on it; talk about it incessantly. Learn to insert your regrets about the past into conversations of all kinds. Never permit the dreadful memory of it to leave you. This will enable you to become a complete flop at present living. Of course you'll become

---

*This term is a combination of Latin, Early American Pig Latin and German. It literally means "before now was not so good."

useless, but you'll have a good reason.

If the guilt gets to you, feel comforted that you have your choice of many psychologists and psychiatrists who will help you by sympathizing with your helplessness in dealing with your miserable past. (Stay away from people who encourage you to move into the present and who will not allow you to let the past paralyze you. These people are problem-robbers and will steal your most carefully developed malady from you unless you remain alert.)

Regret the past and do it persistently, which is sure to make your present counterproductive.

2. The second method is called "basking in the past." The technical term is *"preownaygut."** This approach, also counterproductive, accomplishes basically the same effect on the present as does regretting the past.

It's another way of resting on your laurels through the practice of remembering past glories or remembering the "good old days" to such a degree that you have no time or energy for living in the present.

"Basking in the past" has variations. Examples include: "The present generation is certainly not as good as the children were in our days"; "I remember when things were a lot better in government"; "You sure can't depend on your neighbors like you used to"; "I had such good health back then."

The challenge is to see what a multi-hued, flowering palette you can use to paint your past life events and accomplishments. The more time you spend daydreaming about it, the less time and energy you'll have for useful, productive living in the present. If you (or others) consider your past to be just average in terms of drama and accomplishment, make up things. Embellish! You can make yourself believe if you try hard enough.

3. Method three is commonly called "dreading the future,"

---

*Same etiology as is *preownaynichtgut: preownaygut* literally means "before the present was good."

for which the technical term is *"postownaynichtgut."** This is a stance we can take in the *present* to express cowardice and fear for the *future.*

To accomplish this we need only to imagine the horrors of what *might* happen. Imagine all kinds of calamities ranging from personal ruin to world wars. It is not too difficult. Just remember that nothing is sure and anything can happen. That thought alone, if dwelt upon, can produce king-sized anxieties. It is most important to spend as much of your present time as possible dreading the future. This will assure you of useless-ness in the present and is a built-in excuse for failure. After all, why do anything today when it may all be destroyed in the future?

4. The fourth method is called "dreaming of better days to come." The technical word for this is *"postownaygut."*** This also is a neat counterproductive thought if you over-emphasize it.

Most of the thoughts suggested in this book are true (not all, but most). All of them are, however, useful in producing problems. You see, a thing doesn't have to be erroneous to produce a problem—it just has to be pushed to a counter-productive level. Even good can be used in such a way as to produce evil. One need only look at religious persecutions to learn how effectively truth can be twisted into error. Most heresy is simply truth emphasized to the exclusion of other truths.

If you dream of the future, it will be counterproductive only when you do it to such an extent that you drain off your energy for using the present. Think of all that you are going to do, but never get around to doing it. The idea is to use so much steam blowing the whistle about what is *going to be* that you have none left to power the engine now.

This mode of operation accounts for multitudes of unwritten books, unpainted pictures (and houses), unfinished educations,

---

*Postownaynichtgut literally means "after the present isn't so hot either."
**The literal meaning is "after the present will come the good."

unachieved successes, many unmarried people *and* many married people.

The motto of the counterproductive dreamer of the future is, "Tomorrow, tomorrow, tomorrow, tomorrow or maybe next week!"

The really clever problem-producers can put together the past and future in such a way that they divide their time. They might divide their present thinking time into regretting the past and dreading the future. You do not have to do this in a 50-50 balance. Use whatever is most effective for you.

Those readers who are living useful lives are probably using the bad past as a tool for learning, the good past as encouragement and the future for planning, while focusing on present opportunities or responsibilities. If you wish to lose your health—change your focus. You have a name, too. If you are balancing your life in a productive focus on the present you are among those I call *Zoayownayacs.* *

Zoayownayac is derived from Greek and Early American Pig Latin. It means, "living is for now."

16

Are We Helplessly Helpless?

Helplessness is the stance of all genuine problem-producers from their cradles to their graves. Not only is it the single most important tool of problem-generation, it is also fun to use. If you have been successful in the generation of some maladjustment in your life, you can add a bit of satisfaction for yourself by watching the pained expression on the faces of your mate, friend, therapist, teacher or boss when you say, "and I just can't help it."

No one wants to admit that he/she is responsible for developing personal problems of any kind. It is far more comfortable to project the idea that we are the hapless victims of circumstance or fate. You need not experience the discomfort of responsibility and choice. Even though helplessness is a myth, you do not have to admit it. You only need a few suggestions to *help* you (this is a poor choice of words but I can't help that) hang on to your helplessness.

1. *Never* admit to anyone that you can do better or that you have the power to make personal choices. That is, don't admit it unless you just can't help yourself. In all circumstances insist that you are powerless—totally inadequate to do

anything about your problems. One of my clients liked to point out powerlessness by saying, "There's no use in trying to help me. I am a hopeless case. I've been to therapists and none of them could help me." As of this writing that client's prediction remains true. What a wonderfully frustrating person! You can learn to be equally frustrating with very little practice.

2. Use your imagination and self-talk to convince yourself that the world and every person in your life is enormously powerful and overwhelming in comparison to poor weak little you. After you exaggerate the power of the people in your life, say over and over to yourself, "Now what chance does a weak person like me have against such tremendous odds?" The obvious answer to your question is that you have about as much of a chance of becoming a whole person in this world as you do of dipping all the water out of Lake Michigan with a sieve.

3. Pretend that you are using every ounce of your energy in trying to do something constructive about your problems. Go through the motions of struggling, straining and working hard to overcome whatever problem you have produced for yourself. Periodically you can gasp in exhaustion, "I give up—Oh, God, I just can't do any more."

Lean on anything that will hold your weight and read the following list of opportunities for the use of helplessness. I will give you a starter list of twelve areas where your powerlessness can be utilized as an excuse for your own failures and at the same time drive the people around you into discouraged wrecks.

1. **Temper:** "Oh, I've always had a bad temper. I try to overcome it but there is just no way I can." (Note the use of "always" a beautiful word to use in justifying your present condition.)

2. **Sex:** "I've just never been orgasmic." "I never have been able to last for more than thirty-seven seconds." (Add to the two statements above, "and I never will.") "I have a strong sex drive and one person is never enough for me." "I've just got to have sex at least once each day. It is not my fault, it's just the

way I am."

3. **Fatness:** "I've always been overweight. Everything I eat turns to fat. There is just no way I can lose. I've tried *everything.*" (Notice the double generalizations, "always" and "everything." No one will stop to wonder how anyone could try "everything.")

4. **Depression:** "I never feel up. I am a constantly down person. There is nothing I can do."

5. **Laziness:** "I guess I was just born lazy." (Weren't we all?)

6. **Forgetfulness:** "I have such a bad memory I'd forget my head if it wasn't attached." This gives you an excuse for forgetting birthdays, anniversaries, phone numbers, assignments or going to work.

7. **Drinking or using other drugs:** "You think I want to drink? You've got to be out of your mind. Anyone who could would stay away from this stuff."

8. **Smoking:** "My nerves won't let me quit and besides I've smoked for so long now I'd get physically ill if I tried to quit. I'd give anything if only I could quit."

9. **Tension:** Clench your fist, pop your knuckles, roll your head in a circular motion and bemoan the fact that, "I guess I'm just the type of person who will always be tense."

10. **Nervousness:** "See how my hands shake. I have just had to resign myself to the fact that I will always be nervous."

11. **Stupidity:** Indolence is a warm partner for the cold nights. Who can blame an oaf for making a mess? "Oh, how could I be so dumb? I've been asking myself that since I was four and a half years old."

12. **Filth:** "I'm just sloppy and disorganized. It's the way I am. I can't help it."

No matter what your problem is you can learn to use the language of helplessness. Such language makes it nearly impossible for anyone to take a problem away from you. It isn't very hard to learn. A few key phrases are all you need.

"That's just the way I am."

"It is typical of my sign."

"I am just that type of a person."

"I try, but I can't."

And the key phrase: "I can't help it."

Of course none of these things is true but very few people keep score so they will never know. If you want to give up your problems, you can—because the bitter truth is that *we have a lot of control in our own lives.* I am going to run the risk of illustrating this for you. I know some of you will not like the remainder of this chapter, but I just can't help writing it.

One of the ways I demonstrate to my clients the fact that they have power over their problems is by helping them produce those problems. It is easier to convince a person that he/she is not a helpless victim if he/she sees how effectively anyone can produce depression, anxiety or other malfunction. I call this taking *Negative Control.* You will usually find it easier to begin by producing problems than by solving them.

A few examples will help to illustrate what I mean.

A woman came to me after she had taken an overdose of sleeping pills and tried slashing her wrists with a razor. One might safely conclude that she was very depressed. She was breaking up with her third boy friend. All three relationships had been disastrous for her.

She spoke in a monotone, very softly, shook nervously and cried while talking to me. I asked her how she became depressed. She said she didn't know, and I'm sure that consciously right then she did not.

I suggested that she might imagine, regardless of how ridiculous it sounded, that she wanted to be depressed. I said, "I know you don't want to be—you don't like feeling miserable, but imagine that you do. Is there anything you could do?"

She thought for a moment and said, "Yes, I could call up William. He would tell me to get lost, and that would do it."

"Yes, I imagine it would, but can't you think of something that doesn't involve him directly?" I asked. I knew that rejection from William could be rationalized as something he did to her.

She thought for a more brief time and said, "I could tell

myself how miserable I am without him."

"All right, go on." She was on the right track. This was self-generated.

"I could think of all the good times we had." (This was her misconception. They actually had a miserable relationship, but that didn't matter. The thing that affected her was not reality, but her own perception of it.)

I wondered about other techniques, "How about music? Some people find sad music depressing."

She replied, "Oh, yes. I feel worse when I hear sad music. In fact, I listened to some on the way to your office."

I had learned from other depressed people that they were more depressed when they were alone. I inquired whether this affected her adversely.

She answered, "Yes, I feel worse when I'm alone, and I am alone ninety percent of the time." She began crying more profusely.

I said, "It's all right, go ahead and cry."

She said, "I'm helpless."

I suggested, "Go ahead and be helpless. I'll use what you just told me to help you become more depressed. You might as well have a good one while you are here in my office. Think about the good times you had with William ... think about how miserable you will be without him ... say to yourself that you are helpless and alone. Say over and over to yourself, 'I'm helpless. I'm miserable. Go ahead and feel as depressed as you can.'"

She laughed abruptly, "This is stupid."

I laughed reluctantly, "I didn't mean to mess it up for you but ..."

She interrupted, "... but I'm doing this to myself, and I don't want to. That is stupid."

We then talked for a half hour about more positive, realistic and rational things she could say to herself.

I will illustrate this "helplessness" in two other cases but I could give you dozens of examples almost identical to this one. Before looking at the other examples think of some of the principles involved above.

1. She did this to herself. The therapeutic value of this fact is that if *she* was doing it, she could *stop* doing it. Once she recognized *herself* as being the one in control, she could go either way with her problem.

2. She laughed at herself. The ability to laugh at ourselves is a health-producing agent. We usually take ourselves too seriously.

3. She said negative things to herself. We all talk to ourselves and thus produce most of our feeling responses. Changing what we say to ourselves changes how we feel.

4. I did not try to get her to fight her symptom. A symptom has much more power over us when we fight it than when we just relax about it. Did you ever hear of an insomniac going to sleep by trying to go to sleep? I doubt it. You may have heard of an insomniac going to sleep while trying to wait up for an out-of-town guest. When we stop fighting, we increase our chances for survival. A drowning man flailing at the water will probably drown. He will hamper efforts to rescue him. When he relaxes, he can be helped.

Another example of how "helplessness" is more imagined than real (though it is real to the imaginer) comes from the following encounter with a young woman who had a sexual dysfunction. She could do nothing about it. She was inorgasmic and couldn't help it.

I said, "What I'd like for you to do is not have an orgasm for the next two weeks. Do everything you can to avoid orgasm. When you think it's about to happen, think of something else. Pinch yourself. Do whatever is necessary to avoid it. Then, as soon as the intercourse is finished get up, get a pencil and paper and record for me how you did it. I can use that information to help other people with their sexual problems."

She was a little reluctant. After all, what she really wanted was to have an orgasm. I argued that she wasn't doing that anyway and hadn't for over ten years so she had nothing to lose. Besides, I would help her work on her problem next month. She agreed!

The above took place on Monday. Wednesday I was out of my office in the morning but when I returned my secretary handed me a note. The woman had called. The message she left was, "It happened!" After 10 years of being a helpless victim of her inability to have an orgasm she had had one. The secret? She accepted her helplessness and stopped fighting.

I do not mean to imply that the two people in the foregoing illustrations had solved their problems entirely. They had, however, started in that direction. It will be necessary or at least helpful to work with them in further clarifying their thinking. It will help them to see how they were getting started in problem areas.

A final example of helplessness is a young man who has four girl friends. He is helpless with his own ability to make a decision. All he can do is go from one girl friend to another. He wants to marry one of them, but each one has attributes that made her "the one." He has been in this dilemma for several years.

The beauty of his situation is that he still has four girl friends—all waiting for him to decide while he is helplessly absolved of responsibility. Never mind that no decision is a decision. Never mind that the decision to wait, to procrastinate, is as real as a decision to do something. In his mind and in the minds of his friends, he is a helpless victim of his inability to decide; therefore he is innocent. *He* cannot be responsible because he *wants* to decide; he just can't.

It seems apparent that there are many ways we can use our helplessness. The implication is that we do not have to be helpless. We can make decisions—and in fact, we do decide. If nothing else we decide to use our helplessness. We don't want to face it and we don't want anyone else to know it, but the fact is *we can help our helplessness.*

A Healthy Appendix

The following chapters summarize, in a positive rather than a negative or paradoxical manner, the basic principles upon which the rest of the book is based. The emphasis here is not on how to produce problems, but on how NOT to—or more positively, how to better understand the human in us all. These guidelines, presented with tongue-out-of-cheek and right side up this time, are intended to give people a direction toward healthy and problemless lives.

17

Know These Principles: Make Living Livable

Bankrupt lives, miserable people, battered children, violence, frustration—it's all around me and I ask, "Why?" I have told myself that it is because they just don't know. Ignorance may be bliss for some, but it can be hell for all. People usually don't do better because they don't know better.

There are some principles that you can learn, and by learning them you can make your life better.

1. "Excuse me": We seem to have a tendency to look for excuses. I believe *it is a basic principle of human existence that people actively seek excuses for their problems and behavior.* "I failed the test because I had a headache." "I got drunk because my mother-in-law humiliated me." "I lost the race because the coach overtrained me." "I lost my job because the boss didn't like me."

Excuse-making and excuse-finding probably occupy more of our time and energy than anything we do. If we spent as much time on research as we do on thinking of excuses, we'd probably have discovered a cure for cancer by now. (I probably could have found it myself, but my parents never encouraged me to study science.)

"Gregarious play-person or hermit-like recluse,
One thing we all demand for our behavior is excuse
We do not want shame for it
We do not want blame for it
Ours is to reason and not to die,
We just *have* to tell others the reason why—
I lost my temper, I beat my wife
I cheat on my husband and live a hellish life—
I may be guilty of anything from speeding to assault,
I just try to remember it is someone else's fault."

2. The devil didn't make anybody do it! A second basic principle of human existence is that people really fear responsibility. We fear the responsibility for failure. We fear the responsibility for living. We seek cop-outs through dependency on drugs, work or anything that will enable us to avoid responsibility.

It is our fear of responsibility, the fear that someone will point at us and say, "You are the one who did this," that drives us to our excuse-seeking.

A student who fears failing in school, an athlete who fears being cut from the squad, a person fearing rejection by the opposite sex, a worker who fears losing a job, a spouse who fears failing in marriage or a child who fears displeasing parents—all are potential excuse-seekers.

In a society that has erroneously set up as standards of life such things as material success, approval from others, winning games and prestige, none of us wants to be responsible for even a slight failure. The stupidity in this is that we all do fail from time to time—that's just part of life. We fail and we are responsible. So what's wrong with that? The answer is, "Nothing." We accept responsibility for our own lives, pick up the broken pieces and start over today.

You cannot avoid the responsibility for your own life. In Southeast Missouri we had a saying, "Every tub must sit on its own bottom."

In spite of the impossibility of avoiding responsibility, we all look for excuses—someone to blame. I blame you. You blame me. We both blame our parents, and eventually we blame people from history or someone we made up. When all else fails, we blame Adam, who blamed Eve, who blamed a snake. The devil made us do it!

The fact is, the devil didn't make us do it, we are responsible for our own lives.

3. "I have a goal": When outside excuses fail, we still find a reason for which we cannot be held responsible. We develop an emotional problem or even a physical illness by many of the methods described in this book.

I believe, along with many psychologists (especially Adlerian psychologists), that symptoms have purpose. More often than not, our physical and emotional symptoms have as their purpose enabling us to avoid an unpleasant task, excuse bad behavior or avoid responsibility for failure and losses.

Whether we realize it or not, we generally make use of our emotional or psychological problems. Our symptoms usually have purpose. At times, symptoms are so useful to us that we are reluctant to give them up.

Depression with purpose: We use depression to *gain attention*, reaffirm our importance to significant others, to control others or even to express our pent up hostility. In some situations, depression becomes an excuse for failure.

Some discouraged people believe they are virtually ignored by those around them. They do not have the confidence to believe they can gain attention by "normal" means, so they choose depression as a means to achieve that end. It isn't hard to produce depression, as one may see in the chapter entitled, "The Art of Misery." It is made easier by the belief that no one cares enough about you to listen or pay attention to you. Whether by accident or by design, you quickly learn that people sit up and take notice if you become depressed. This is doubly reinforced when you talk about or threaten suicide. Gaining attention is not always, or even usually, a conscious action, but it is frequently the purpose.

It is easy to see how added attention from other people in your life can reaffirm your importance. If they care enough to pay attention or try to help you overcome your depression, then you must be important to them.

Gaining control is a more subtle, but probably a prominent, use of depression. A depressed mate can keep a spouse from going out to participate in social activities or recreation. Again, this may happen because the depressed person is discouraged and afraid to participate in activities outside the home.

Another form of control is the *inducement of guilt* in the people around you. When this is the purpose, the depressed person may imply or directly state, "It's your fault that I feel this way," or, "If it weren't for you I'd feel better." This may result in the accused working harder to keep his or her depressed friend, mate or family member from feeling bad. The efforts are usually to no avail!

Perhaps the most obvious use of or purpose for depression is the *expression of pent-up hostility*. This use becomes clear when we see the ultimate depression in total withdrawal (the refusal to communicate, as in a pouting, angry child) or in suicide—an obvious act of hostility. Frequently the purpose becomes transparent when we find suicide notes that say things like, "Now you'll realize how much you hurt me," "This will show them how important I was," "Maybe they'll miss me now." To leave behind a person living with blame or guilt with no chance to make amends is a super act of anger or hostility.

Such acts result when people either do not know how to express hostility, have been discouraged when they try to express anger or have been afraid to express it.

One of my clients was just learning how to express her anger. Her husband had been told of our efforts to teach her to express anger openly because she had already attempted suicide. In spite of these precautions, he instinctively responded with violence when the client openly expressed her anger to him. He did not want her to express anger toward him. He used his power to get her out of therapy. The tragic ending to this story is that after a brief hospitalization this former client successfully attempted suicide. She had finally expressed anger and no one could retaliate.

This brief example indicates how we sometimes inadvertently push a depressed person back into a pattern with which they feel more comfortable. They may decide again that the only way they can "safely" express their anger is through their deep depression.

One final example of the uses of depression is *as an excuse for our failures*. The courage to fail is a rare virtue in human beings. We usually want to find an excuse.

In Chapter 3, I mentioned some of the basic causes of depression. It is interesting to list them along side the hypothesized uses or purposes of depression.

Causes	Purposes
Feelings of unworthiness	Gain attention
	Reaffirm importance
	Control
Guilt and failure	Excuses
Repressed hostility	Expressing hostility

The implication for the layman, as well as the therapist, is that if we use our depression we must be able to produce it or sustain it. In other words, we do control our emotions, at least in many situations. It also stands to reason that if we produce them, we may also overcome them.

Anger with purpose: We use anger for a lot of reasons.

1. We can use anger *to make people around us do what we want them to do*. Many a husband or wife has been heard to say, "I'd better not do that," or "I'd better do this," then add, "because it will make my spouse angry if I do (or don't)." We train our spouses, children, employer, employees or peers to do what we want done by holding the threat of our anger over them.

2. We sometimes use our anger *to get attention or get*

someone to listen. "I have to yell and throw things before they will listen to me."

Certainly we do not want to admit that we have control of our temper, so we fall back on helplessness. We speak of ourselves as having bad tempers. We speak of temper as if it were a disease we have because of our descent, our red hair, our environment, our size or a malfunction of our nerves. We sound like victims. "I can't help it. I've just got a terrible temper." We usually want people to interpret that claim as "my terrible temper has got me."

The fallacy of our claim to be helpless victims can be clearly seen. If you are "caught" by your terrible temper and are in the midst of a screaming, swearing, stomping "fit" and a distinguished guest rings the door bell it is amazing to note the speed with which you regain control. (I say "regain," but really believe it is simply exercising control in another direction.) I have caught myself doing this. I have been in the middle of a severe seizure by my temper when the phone has rung. I am somewhat embarrassed when I note the gentle tone of my voice as I say, "Hello."

It would be impossible to guess how many uncontrollable tempers, causing terrible fights, have been cooled by the ringing of a school bell that signaled the end of recess.

We certainly have more control than we exercise, and thus I believe we use our tempers to achieve our purposes at the moment.

Self-pity and tears with purpose: Tears are often used in the same way. (I am not suggesting that we forbid expressions of anger or stop crying, but I am suggesting that we would be more honest to admit control more often than we usually do.)

I have seen clients use crying as a tool. This was clearly seen with a couple I saw last year. They were having what they considered to be serious marital problems. She could listen to him talk, but everytime she tried to talk, she cried. I was beginning to feel uncomfortable, so I said to her, "You sure cry a lot, don't you?"

Her husband answered for her, "Oh, God, does she ever! I can't discuss a problem with her for fear that she will cry."

Their marriage honestly began to turn around and grow when she stopped "using" her tears. She was using tears to avoid conflict, but her cure was far worse than the disease. The fact is that her tears were adding a great deal to their problems.

It will certainly come as no shocking revelation to most of you that we use our tears to gain sympathy for ourselves. "If they see me crying, they'll know how hurt I really am." Ironically, again, the tool often works against us. Instead of achieving its intended purpose, it can actually irritate people, especially if used to excess.

It can be seen that we also use our laughter to conceal feelings. The point I'm making is not that it is "bad" to use our emotions or symptoms. The point is that we can and do use them. This may be uncomfortable because it demands that we face our behaviors responsibly, but it is also encouraging. I am glad that I have a lot of control over my emotions. We all have a goal.

4. "I have decided": Not only do we use our symptoms to excuse ourselves from responsibility, we have a great deal more control over them than we are usually comfortable enough to admit. In a very real and at times most powerful sense we often *choose* our symptoms.

The fourth principle of human existence is that human beings are creatures of choice. We have more choice than any other animal. We may push choices into our subconscious actions, or we may call them forth consciously. We are free to choose. It seems to me that people hide from the responsibility of choice by saying, "I can't." It would be more accurate to say, "I do not choose to ..." "I can't" is helpless, while "I choose" comes from a position of strength and control.

We can choose to be happy, to enjoy life or to be miserable. "Oh, but," you say, "we cannot control the circumstances of life and death." It is true that we cannot control circumstances, but we can control stance. We determine the attitude we take toward our circumstances. It is like being dealt a hand of cards in a poker game. We do not determine what cards we get, but we decide how to play the hand!

I have learned that I can choose to control my temper.

5. **"Any fool can see this. Why, I see it"**: One reason that it is hard for us to recognize the control, production and use of our emotions is our ability to rationalize. The fifth principle of human existence is our ability to use what Adlerians call "private logic."

We all develop some forms of tunnel vision. We filter what we hear, what we see, what we do and what we remember through our own private screens. It is quite natural because we are always gathering data as evidence that prove our views to be correct, our expectations to be fulfilled and our behavior to be justified.

A young man came to me saying he believed his wife was being sexually unfaithful to him. He told himself that he was inadequate as a husband, that he had never been able to please her, even though she told him otherwise. He said no one could love someone like him. His wife agreed to come for counseling with him. She said that she cared a great deal for him but that she could not convince him.

I asked him how she could prove that she loved him and didn't want anyone else. He, of course, didn't know. I pointed out to him that even if she swore and signed a notarized affidavit, it would not be enough. The fact is that unless we are willing to believe we are loved and accepted, there is no way anyone can prove it to us.

This young man's private logic was foolproof. He was "no good." He could not please any woman because he was not a "real" man. Given these ideas he could only conclude: "Therefore my wife cannot love me." Unless he can change his concept of himself, he will never be able to believe he is loved. Life does not come with written guarantees.

There are many times that we simply do not see or hear the

things that disagree with our own views. This tendency makes it almost impossible for us to view our own lives or world objectively. This is the reason that it is more difficult for us to evaluate and understand our own behavior than that of anyone else. "Well, it certainly made sense to me." "Of course I know I am right."

I have been frustrated when I have clearly made statements concerning the equality of men and women and the equality of the races, only to have someone who had filtered my words through their own private screens say to me that I totally ignored the issue of equality. On some of those occasions, I had the good fortune of having tapes of what I said. My biased listeners were embarrassed to hear what was actually said.

I believe we all do basically the same kind of selective listening and observing. This explains how we can use symptoms and even produce them with purpose without being aware of our actions.

6. "Woe is me": A sixth basic principle of human existence is that human beings are so afraid and prejudiced against themselves that they are easily discouraged. This is the reason that criticism is so useless in trying to help a person change. Discouraged people misbehave, become defensive and lock into their private logic concerning their purposes.

Three very clear examples of discouraging words or ideas will make it apparent that we are easily discouraged and that discouragement is useless. Think of how you react to criticism, rejection and fear.

One of the most powerful instruments of discouragement is, or course, criticism. We are never able to help people overcome their problems by criticizing them. All we do is discourage them (note chapter on "Walling the Generation Gap"). Parents mistakenly think they are helping their children when they criticize them; in truth, they are discouraging them. Some people think they are helping their spouses when they criticize them; in truth, they are discouraging them.

Criticism does not help people to change; it hinders them.

Another instrument of discouragement is *rejection*. All that is said of criticism can be said of rejection. People with problems are usually discouraged, and to criticize or reject them just further discourages them.

The counterpart of rejection is *acceptance*. Acceptance of the person regardless of his or her problem is an instrument of encouragement. This book is an attempt to communicate acceptance of people regardless of their problems and thus to become an instrument of encouragement.

My friends Bill and Mim Pew say, "No one has ever died of too much encouragement." It would be wonderful if we could start a movement based on encouragement.

Fear is both an instrument of discouragement and a principle of human life. Fear of failure, fear of rejection and even fear of death all cause people to retreat from conflict resolution, from confrontation with life and from problem-solving in general. Alfred Adler said that fear is the greatest enemy of cooperation and that social cooperation is essential to problem-solving. It is my hope that by reducing problems to the absurd we can reduce their capacity to produce fear.

7. "You can't make me do it": A seventh basic principle of human nature is contrariness. Human beings are perverse and stubborn creatures. We do not like to be told what to do, and very often we rebel. It is the reason that "reverse psychology" frequently works. It is clearly illustrated in the story of Brer Fox and Brer Rabbit. The rabbit pleaded not to be thrown in the briar patch, which was precisely the thing he desired. The fox, not being skilled in psychology, fell for the trick and threw the rabbit in the briar patch.

Very often this trait shows up when we ask a client to do something. He or she resists. Many of us who like Adlerian principles have learned to stop fighting and even prescribe the symptom.

On more than one occasion, I have asked a client to recount an early recollection, something that happened before he or she was seven years old. When the client can remember nothing, if I then say, "All right, make up a story about what might have happened to you," he or she somehow remembers the previously forgotten material. This is a mild form of contrariness. There is a little rebel in all of us. I see it every day in my office, and I sense it every day in my own life. When I'm told not to do something, there is a feeling of rebellion that begins to gnaw at me. That same feeling occurs when I'm told I must do something. Perhaps it is an innate drive to be free to choose. I do not know. All I know is that it is there.

It is that contrariness in all of us which may help us to conquer problems that we are told to produce. At least it demonstrates our power over our problems.

It is my hope that we can fall back on our basic reasonableness and see that, underneath it all, we are rational creatures who can overcome most of the obstacles that hinder us from reaching our goals of adjustment and peace within ourselves.

Human contrariness is what makes paradoxical intention work in counseling.

8. "Want Power": Human beings most often do what they want to do. I frequently hear people talk about their will power or lack of will power. Clients say things like, "I would stop smoking but I just can't. I don't have the will power.

I responded to a client who made that statement by asking, "Do you think you could stop smoking if I paid you ten dollars a day for not smoking?"

The client paused and said, "I doubt it."

I suggested, "For one hundred dollars a day?"

There was a longer pause, "I don't know."

I raised the ante, "Could you quit if I paid you a thousand dollars a day for not smoking?"

There was no pause, "You bet I could!"

I said, "Well, quit then."

A smile came to the lips of the client, "Will you give me a thousand dollars a day?"

I was honest, "Of course not."

The client stopped smiling, "I'd like to, but I can't."

I dropped the bomb, "We've already established that you *can*—it's just a matter of price now. If you are motivated enough you can. You have the will power. You just don't have the want power."

You can apply this basic principle to many areas of discipline: overeating, drinking, other dependencies, control of temper or using time to work or study. Try it on yourself. Could you do whatever you think you can't do if the price were high enough? If so, you are probably experiencing a deficiency in *want power*.

It is a basic principle of human life that people have about as much will power as they want to use.

9. "The laugh is on me": A ninth basic principle of human nature is that people take themselves too seriously. Most of what I have written in this book is designed to help us stop taking ourselves too seriously. I have discovered that many very serious problems become funny when we look at them objectively. Most people seem to know this instinctively. We frequently hear people say, "If you could only see yourself you would laugh."

Though it is often a tragic humor, life *is* filled with humor. If most married couples could see their fights or arguments acted out on stage, they would see them as hilariously funny.

The same is true of individual behaviors. If we could see the way we defeat ourselves by giving in to symptoms, holding onto erroneous ideas or wading up to our whatever in self-pity, we would laugh.

The need for an ability to laugh at ourselves is apparent when we see how problems lose their power in the presence of honest humor. When we laugh at a problem it loses its power over us.

I am suggesting that:

1. People, all of us, seek excuses for our problems and behavior;

2. We are actually responsible for our own emotions, problems and behavior in almost all circumstances;
3. Emotions, problems and human behavior have purpose;
4. We have the power to choose control in our own lives;
5. We rationalize our own behavior and problems by using private logic;
6. Human beings are basically biased against themselves;
7. We are all, at least a little bit, contrary or stubborn;
8. We have about as much will power as we want;
9. We take ourselves too seriously most of the time.

18

Tying It All Together

We can all live with less tension and more confidence. We can learn to feel better about ourselves. This can be accomplished if we begin with the admission that we are responsible for our own lives. At first I don't mind tension, illness or failure if I do not have to accept responsibility for it, if it is not my fault. However, the more that I reflect on my "fate," the more discouraged I become.

"Must I continue to be a victim?"

"Am I just a mechanical response to the external stimuli around me?"

The encouraging truth is that I am not a victim. I am not a helpless mechanical response. I am a human being who has a choice about and responsibility for my own life, and I'm damned tired of being told otherwise by psychologists, psychiatrists, clergymen, astrologers and, too often, the media.

The principles written in this book are just negative ways— and hopefully humorous ways—of illustrating the control and choice we have in our own lives. These principles suggest that we not only can, but do, create problems and even sicknesses for ourselves.

I hope the reader has been "paradoxed" by this book. By being paradoxed, I mean that if you have any of the problems mentioned in this book I hope I have successfully put my wind into your sails. I hope you have been able to say, "Hey, that's what I do. I must be producing problems for myself. I am going to stop it, now!"

If you have been using your symptoms as excuses or to teach goals, I hope I have "spit in your soup"* so that you will no longer want to eat it. You can choose more courageous ways of dealing with failures and other problems and of reaching your goals.

I will summarize briefly some thoughts that will tie all these concepts together and will enable you to live more courageously and usefully for yourself and others.

First, *consciously acknowledge the fact that your life is filled with choices.* When you are confronted with situations that may be used to generate fear, depression, anger, tension, say to yourself confidently and repeatedly "I have a choice. I can choose to turn this situation into an opportunity to grow in courage, strengthen my base for happiness, demonstrate my patience and power, and become more relaxed about life."

Second, *consciously and deliberately choose to accept responsibility for your own behavior and life.* Decide now to stop hiding behind circumstances, fate or any symptoms you may have. Stop blaming your background, your family, your job or anything outside yourself for your own attitudes and life. Say to yourself and to others, "I am responsible for my anger. I can choose to use it or to control it. I do with my emotions and my life basically what I want to do."

I am contrary enough that I resent it when others tell me I am responsible for my behavior, but in my more honest moments I admit that it is true. It feels a lot better to me when I tell myself that I am responsible. Try it. It feels good!

---

*Alfred Adler called anti-suggestion or directing a person toward their symptoms "spitting in their soup."

Third, *consciously choose to live from a position of strength.* I talk to a lot of people who live and act from a position of weakness. They say things like: "I am afraid to do that, I might not be able to succeed"; "I am afraid to say that because people might not like me if I did"; "I can't say or do what I would really like because my wife or husband wouldn't love me."

Even if you do the best things but do them from a position of weakness, they lose their value to you. You can choose to live from a position of strength if you are willing to pay the price. Face your fears. Face people and situations you fear. Stop running afraid!

When you take this courageous stance, you will approve of yourself. You will learn that you can even love yourself. It seems to me that loving yourself and approving of yourself is the only base from which your love for others and approval of others has any real value.

Fourth, *consciously choose to find your own meaning in life.* If your life has no meaning to you, it is your own responsibility. You can choose to do and be the things that have meaning to you.

I have found meaning for my life in my commitment to Jesus Christ. It is my responsible decision. I do not try to force my belief on anyone else. I respect your right to choose whatever faith you want, or no faith at all—that is your responsibility.

For many years I lived my life as I thought other Christians expected me to live it. It meant very little. I then became "intellectual" and let the other "intellectuals" influence my acts and words. I became reluctant to share my basic beliefs.

I have more recently discovered that the real religionists and the real intellectuals do not mutually exclude one another and that I can choose to be honest with both groups. I find my meaning through my faith and commitment to God. Find yours, and accept the responsibility for your choice. Do not permit theological or psychological bullies to push you around. Find your own meaning.

Fifth, *consciously choose to remind yourself that life is for now.* You may plan as if you will live forever, but always live as if today is all you have, because it is.

The encouraging thing about life being for now is that we only have to live it one day at a time. It was Jesus who said that each day's evil is sufficient in and of itself. If you focus on life today, you do have the power to live it.

Learn to accept life in smaller pieces. You can't eat a whole meal with one gulp, so you eat it one bite at a time. A book isn't written with one movement of the pen. It is written one word—one letter—at a time. Life is lived one day at a time.

You can accept almost anything when you realize it is only for this day.

Finally, *I suggest that you consciously choose to enjoy your life.* Life is filled with many things that are fun, but enjoyment is beyond fun and games. I do not believe you will always be privileged to do what you enjoy, but I do believe you have the power to choose to enjoy most of what you do.

Don't be afraid to laugh at yourself. As a matter of fact, why don't you take a good look at yourself today and say, "You are a nice person and I like you because you do so many funny things."

We have a choice. We have immense power within us. We can overcome problems, or if we want a problem we can produce one.

The choice is yours. Why don't you drive yourself sane?

19

Making the Best Use Of This Book

Look for Balance

Fanatics: Someone has defined a fanatic as a person who, having lost sense of direction, redoubles his or her effort. It seems to me that a lot of self-help writers and readers have lost their sense of direction. The result is that fanatics scream from radio programs, television programs, newspapers and books, "Do this and you will live better." The more confused the cry, the faster they run.

Turning truth into a lie: It has also been said that truth pushed to an exclusive position can become a lie. Even when people begin with truth, they can become liars if they lose their balance.

When you read a book such as this one, you become responsible for maintaining balance. Even the valid principles (and most of mine are) can be pushed to a place where they are not only no longer helpful but can be harmful.

For example, in general the Beasley Principle is valid and helpful, but if you use that principle to avoid all responsibility for the effect of your behavior on the rest of society, it becomes a socially (thus personally) useless principle. Total irresponsibility says, "I'll do what I want, you do what you want, and it doesn't matter to either of us." A society of such people would be a society of spoiled brats at best and sociopaths at worst.

You are responsible for your own balance: The truth is in *balance*. We are all responsible for our own behavior, but we are not so stupid as to believe that none of our behavior effects other people. If you push principles to illogical conclusions, you could become a thief and steal posessions from others and then rationalize, "That's not my problem." When this is done, a healthy concept becomes a sick concept.

It becomes then, your responsibility to maintain balance in your own life and in your own marriage. Certainly individuality is important. Personal growth is vital. Personal freedom is tremendously important. The point is that healthy individuality, healthy personal freedom and healthy personal growth do not exclude—rather they *include*—responsible behavior toward and with other people.

Goals: It is not my goal, nor do I believe it is the goal of other self-help writers, to create selfish people who run around ignoring the rights of others and behaving in socially irresponsible ways. It is my hope that by becoming a stronger, growing individual you will become a more creative, significant contributor to your own family and social world.

Balance of dependence and independence from historical perspectives: Without becoming too philosophical, I want to share my opinion of what has happened historically. We are influenced by the movement of history, and we went through a period of rugged individualism and isolationism in pioneer America. We, as a nation, moved to the opposite extreme after World War I and took on the problems of the world. Everyone was given encouragement for expressing concern.

During the first period, we adapted the individual spirit to our own lives, and each person did his or her own thing. It was not effective, so we moved, along with the nation, to the other extreme of concern for one another in an ever shrinking world.

From calloused individual selfishness, we moved to self-defeating overconcern. (A practice as detrimental to persons as nuclear overkill is to the world.) We are now experiencing the swing of the pendulum back to self-fulfillment. The battle cry becomes, "Do your own thing! Let each person fend for himself or herself."

I have the nagging hunch that we are moving toward imbalance again. My hypothesis is that the most healthy position is one that blends together personal responsibility and personal freedom. They are not mutually exclusive concepts. You can determine the amount of concern for social responsibility you are comfortable handling, while at the same time assuming the freedom to choose responsibly your own life style. All I'm saying is that life is not lived in a vacuum, and we do depend on one another.

Healthy dependence coupled with healthy independence evolves into mutual interdependence, which is an essential for the continued existence of democracy—and families.

Free and responsible: Think of the implications of either extreme. On the one end, there are those people who are totally dependent on the attitudes and reactions of others for their sense of security and value. If you fall into this group, you can spend your whole life never knowing what you could become or even what you are. And that is nonsense!

On the other extreme are those people who want to live for themselves only. They say *my* drinking, *my* sexual expressions, *my* behavior has nothing to do with the rest of the world or, for that matter, anyone else. Such isolationism is also nonsense!

The Key: The key is balance, and balance is something you can and will discover for yourself.

Apply It to Yourself

The hazard: The other hazard in writing a self-help book is that a good many readers will see it as a book that "someone I know needs to read." Good! Share it with as many people as you can, but please remember that "self-help" is most effectively applied by self to self.

For an example: I still do not like someone else to tell me I am responsible for my behavior. I feel a lot better about the whole process if I can tell myself I am responsible. That is not nearly so threatening.

Result of misapplication: What happens when you start applying these principles to others? The thing that usually happens is that they will feel threatened, thus they will be defensive.

You can only change yourself: Defensiveness closes the mind so in the final analysis you defeat your own purposes. Remember this. The only person you have the power and the responsibility to change is you. So apply the principles to yourself.

Drive yourself sane. And then share your experience and how it works for you and let others assume responsibility for themselves!

20

Postscript

Letter from a Client who Applied some of these Principles

"Dear Bill:

The former me was a void. There was nothing positive, creative, or substantial about her. She was totally empty of the ability to feel, act, or interact. Like any space, she was limited and shaped by things surrounding her, formed by things outside her. She was passive; she felt helpless and hopeless. Ennui and a feeling of total uselessness caused deep depression. While she existed, she did not 'live' in real terms. Today, looking back on her, I still vividly feel her pain and fear, but each day I find it more difficult to relate to her and identify with her. This separation from her was gradual. While I was going to you, when people told me I had changed I was very defensive. Today I consider the same comment a compliment.

(I have a choice) "The real me of today *is*. I know that sounds like an incomplete idea, but actually it is the way I see myself. I am—I'm an energy, a force, a being, a reality! Even though

I've been the new me for almost six months, the sense of power is still pretty heady. I guess one of the reasons I find it difficult to define myself now is because I haven't decided what I'm going to be yet. Before I didn't think I could be anything. Today I have so many options, I find it difficult to make decisions. It's all so new.

(I can laugh at myself) "I also find myself amusing and fun. I mean, here I am, at thirty, experiencing for the first time what most children or adolescents are accustomed to. Much of it is frightening, but it is also so new that it is fun. Life is kind of like a grand adventure. *Each day*, and I mean that literally, I learn something new about me or the world. (It's really ironic that you asked me to write this at this time, because I really do identify with Easter and the whole theme of rebirth.)

"Now comes the hard part, that third question. What did you do to help me in our sessions? I know that for the purpose of your book you'd like me to list specific aspects of the psychology that were most helpful to me, but I find this impossible to do without dealing with it in a larger concept. If it had not been for your caring and your offer of friendship at our initial session, I'm not sure how effective the rest of the sessions would have been. One of my most vivid remembrances of our sessions is what you said at that first session. You said you liked me. To be honest, that floored me. I remember being puzzled as to what you liked. Then when you asked me if I liked you, I was impressed by the risk you were taking. What if I said no? But it was your next comment that really struck. When I said yes, you said that it didn't mean much because I was incapable of disliking anybody. I think it was then that you told me I was a worthwhile human being and didn't have to do anything or be anything to prove that. Having been raised in a highly Christian environment, I had heard that many times. But this was the first time I had it correctly practiced on me.

"You were also very positive that you could help me at that session, but I wasn't convinced. The real reason I came back was that I liked the fact that you cared and I trusted you.

"This idea of self-worth was really the most important help you gave me. First, you told me I didn't have to do anything I didn't want to. I still laugh when I think how hard it was for me to accept this idea. Now it's my first commandment. Every morning I ask myself if I really want to go to work. Every day I decide I really want to. Since I've been doing that, I actually enjoy my job.

"Second, you convinced me to be honest with people. If I give them anything but the real me, I'm going to end up hurting them or disappointing them. This idea has removed a lot of the pressure I used to feel in dealing with people. Now I just act myself and people are free to accept or reject that.

(**Beasley principles**) "That was the third 'biggie' I learned in therapy, Beasleyism. I only deal with my own problems now. This really helps me keep things in perspective. I don't try to do the impossible anymore.

"The second important help you gave me was confidence. Once you convinced me that even if I did fail at something I would still survive, risks didn't seem so overwhelming. This became an obsessive idea. I started giving myself all sorts of little dares just to see if I could do them. I'll have you know that I've even attempted parallel parking.

"Another thing that helped build this confidence was when we talked about wants and needs. Once I got these things into perspective, I felt life was making much fewer demands of me. My needs were pretty easy to meet. I've got millions of wants, but now I see them for what they are, icing on the cake. I'm now confident I can deal with life's little (and big) problems because they are just that, problems—not life or death situations.

"The third important help you gave me was sexuality. I can now accept this in me. I'm not confused about the role I want to play sexually. I enjoy being a woman. I enjoy being thinner and take pains with how I look. I'm not threatened when men find me attractive. I'm actually anxious to find a meaningful relationship with a man and be able to express myself sexually. But, even if this never happens, my awareness and acceptance of my sexuality makes me happy with myself.

"I like myself!"

About the Author

Bill L. Little, a native of Gideon, Missouri, holds a B.A. from East Texas Baptist College, a Th.M. from Midwestern Baptist Theological Seminary, an M.S. from Southern Illinois University, and a Ph.D. from Washington University.

For over thirty years, he has been pastor of Christ Memorial Baptist Church in St. Louis. For over twenty, he has been a professional therapist. Since 1977 he has been known to a wide radio audience for his on-the-air counseling over station KMOX, St. Louis. He has been team psychologist for two baseball teams—the St. Louis Cardinals from 1980-82, and the Seattle Mariners from 1983-87—using visualization techniques to help improve sports performance. He has taught at Washington University, University of Missouri in St. Louis, and Missouri Baptist College, and has conducted conferences on alcoholism marriage and family relations, stress communications, management and motivation.

He is the author of ˙ Help Yourself Heal (CompCare) and several magazine articles.

www.ingramcontent.com/pod-product-compliance
Lightning Source LLC
Chambersburg PA
CBHW030012290326
41934CB00005B/309